Fannie Rutt's
MURPH WORKOUT GUIDE

Military-Style Training Guide With Proven Strategies, Workout Regimes, and Motivations That Will Set You on a Path for Success and Supercharge Your Performance!

FANNIE RUTT

TABLE OF CONTENTS

Introduction

Millions of individuals train out daily all around the globe but are not seeing the expected results. They were duped by out-of-date rules of thumb, misleading promises about diet or training techniques, or just plain stupid bro-science. Many of us were taught that if we do X, Y will follow. And if it still hasn't happened, keep pressing until the desired outcomes appear. As an experienced personal trainer, believe me when I say this: if it hasn't worked for you up to this point, your program will never bring you to your gym objectives. Everyone is unique: we have different metabolisms, limb-torso ratios, muscle attachment sites; our hormone systems work differently, and we don't even have the same muscles! To begin, everyone has a unique ratio of slow-twitch and rapid twitch muscle fibres, which determines whether you are more likely to gain bulk quickly or whether you are more likely to remain lean. Second, some muscles are only present in specific individuals (e.g. plantaris muscle, psoas minor muscle). So, chances are you'll have to experiment a lot before you discover the exercises, methods, and rest periods that have the potential to truly help you accomplish your gym objectives - whether it's greater strength, more bulk, overall athleticism, or just developing a more appealing body. The only established technique for progress is to test, apply, and then test again. Simply said, there are too many.

There are many factors to consider! So far, science has done an excellent job of describing various body systems and how they respond to various kinds of training, but in each research, only a few factors can be controlled. When you exercise, dozens, if not hundreds, of factors interact in a complicated manner to produce a specific metabolic response to your training session.

This book is mainly aimed at experienced lifters and individuals who have been exercising at home for at least a year. The majority of everything you will read will require a solid physical basis. If you're searching for fresh ways to break past plateaus, this book will provide you with additional choices. More choices for working on hypertrophy, more possibilities for squeezing in a short exercise on the fly, more options for working on strength and recovery. If your exercise theory hasn't produced the results you've been hoping for, be prepared to turn it on its head. Be curious enough to try out some totally new training methods. Be ready to try new things and abandon them if they don't work - but at least give it a fair go for six to eight weeks. Be all of that, but don't trust anything I say! Be open to new ideas inside and outside of the gym, and believe in what works for you! Work, sweat, repeat...and enjoy the process!

THE MASS CARDS (THE 101 MASS CARDS)

First-Placed Card

MONDAY

Chest and biceps exercises

Chest:

- 3 sets of 15 chest presses. Obtain a minute.
- 3 sets of 15 dip machines Obtain a minute.
- Crosses to the wires in three groups of fifteen. Obtain a minute.

biceps:

- 3x15 curl cable I'm looking for a minute.
- 3x15 arm carl machine I'm looking for a minute.
- 3 × 15-minute recovery curl to the wires over the head

WEDNESDAY'
Workout for the Shoulders and Legs
Shoulder blades:
- 3 sets of 15 shoulder presses I'm looking for a minute.
- Rope side risers or a 3x15 machine I'm looking for a minute.

legs:
- 3x15 Leg Extensions I'm looking for a minute.
- Press 3x15. I'm looking for a minute.

- 3 sets of 15 leg curls I'm looking for a minute.
- 3x20 calf standing, I'm looking for a minute.

FRIDAY'

Dorsal and triceps exercises

backbone:

- 3x15 wide grip lat machine I'm looking for a minute.
- 3x15 pulley down tight Grip I'm looking for a minute.
- 3x15 Lat Machine Tight Grip I'm looking for a minute.

Triceps:

- Triceps cables (rail) 3x15 wide Grip I'm looking for a minute.

- Triceps cables with strong grip ropes 3x15 I'm looking for a minute.

- CARD is ranked second.

-WORKOUT 02

MONDAY'

- Chest and biceps exercises

Chest:

- 3 sets of 10 chest presses. Obtain a minute.
- 3 sets of 10 dip machines Obtain a minute.
- Butterfly machine with three sets of ten. Obtain a minute.

biceps:

- 3x10 curl cable I'm looking for a minute.
- 3x10 arm carl machine I'm looking for a minute.
- 3 x 10 curls to the wires over the head. I'm looking for a minute.

WEDNESDAY'

- Workout for the Shoulders and Legs

Shoulder blades:

- 3 sets of 10 shoulder presses I'm looking for a minute.
- Rope side risers or a 3x10 machine I'm looking for a minute.

legs:

- 3x10 Leg Extension I'm looking for a minute.
- 3x10 print. I'm looking for a minute.
- 3 sets of 10 leg curls I'm looking for a minute.
- 3x10 calf sitting I'm looking for a minute.

FRIDAY'

Dorsal and triceps exercises
backbone:
- 3x10 wide grip lat machine I'm looking for a minute.
- 3x10 pulley down tight Grip I'm looking for a minute.
- 3x10 Lat Machine Tight Grip I'm looking for a minute.

Triceps:

- Triceps cables (rail) 3x10 wide Grip I'm looking for a minute.
- Triceps cables with strong grip ropes 3x10. I'm looking for a minute.
- CARD is ranked third.

-WORKOUT 03

MONDAY'

Chest and biceps exercises

Chest:

- 4 sets of 6 chest presses I'm looking for a minute.
- 4 sets of 6 dip machines I'm looking for a minute.
- Crosses to the wires in three groups of ten. Obtain a minute.

biceps:
- 4x6 curl cable I'm looking for a minute.
- Carl machine 4x6 arm. I'm looking for a minute.
- 3 x 8 curl to the wires over the head. I'm regaining a minute.

WEDNESDAY'

Workout for the Shoulders and Legs

Shoulder blades:

- 4x6 shoulder press I'm looking for a minute.
- Rope side risers or a 3x10 machine I'm looking for a minute.

legs:

- Leg press 4x8. I'm looking for a minute.
- 3x8 Leg Extension I'm looking for a minute.
- 3x8 Leg Curls I'm looking for a minute.
- 3x8 calf sitting I'm looking for a minute.

FRIDAY'

- Dorsal and triceps exercises

backbone:

- 4x6 Lat Machine Wide Grip I'm looking for a minute.
- 3x6 pulley down tight Grip I'm looking for a minute.
- 3x8 Lat Machine Tight Grip I'm looking for a minute.

Triceps:

- Triceps cables (rail) 3x8 wide Grip I'm looking for a minute.
- Triceps cables with a 3x8 strong grip. I'm looking for a minute.
- -Card ranked fourth

-WORKOUT 04

MONDAY'

Chest and biceps exercises

Chest:

- 3 sets of 8 chest presses with a broad grip I'm regaining a minute.
- 3 sets of 8 chest presses with a tight grip. I'm regaining a minute.
- Crosses to the wires in three groups of twelve. Obtain a minute.

biceps:

- 6 + 6 + 6 + 6 + 6 + 6 + 6 + 6 I'm getting a minute and a half.
- Strip cables 3x 6 + 6 + 6 curling. I'm getting a minute and a half.

WEDNESDAY'

- Workout for the Shoulders and Legs
- Shoulder blades:
- 3x6 + 6 + 6 shoulder press stripping I'm getting a minute and a half.
- Rope side risers or a 3x8 vehicle I'm looking for a minute.

legs:

- Stripping press machine 3x6 + 6 + 6. I'm getting a minute and a half.
- 3x12 Leg Extension I'm looking for a minute.
- 3 sets of 12 leg curls I'm looking for a minute.
- 3x12 calf sitting I'm looking for a minute.

FRIDAY'

- Dorsal and triceps exercises

backbone:

- 3x10 superset of lat machine wide grip pulldowns with tight grip pulldowns. I'm getting a minute and a half.
- 3x10 pulley down tight Grip I'm looking for a minute.

Triceps:

- Triceps cables (rail) 4x6 broad Grip I'm looking for a minute.
- Triceps cables with a 4x6 strong grip. I'm looking for a minute.

- CARD is ranked 5th.

-WORKOUT 05

MONDAY'

Exercise your chest and triceps.

Chest:

Stripping sequence 6 + 6 + 6 on the chest push 3 (It begins with a heavy weight to create six, then decreases the weight on the next and even the next to complete the final six.) I'm getting a minute and a half.
- 3 sets of 8 dip machines I'm regaining a minute.
- Crosses to the wires in three groups of twelve. Obtain a minute.

Triceps:

- Triceps cables 3x12 great reverse Grip I'm looking for a minute.
- Triceps cables 3x12 with ropes strong Grip I'm looking for a minute.

WEDNESDAY'

- Workout for the Shoulders and Legs

Shoulder blades:

- 4x8 shoulder press I'm looking for a minute.
- Rope side risers or 3x6 car + 6 + 6 stripping I'm getting a minute and a half.

legs:

- With the leg extension, do a super sequence of presses. 4x8. four press series and four
- Extensions of the legs Basically, it's an 8-rep set followed by an 8-rep restless sequence of presses

before switching to leg extensions for another 8 reps. Rest for one and a half minutes.

- 3 sets of 10 leg curls I'm looking for a minute.
- 3x10 calf sitting I'm looking for a minute.

FRIDAY'

- Training and biceps latissimusdorsi.

backbone:

- Stripping socket for Lat Machine 3x6 + 6 + 6. I'm getting a minute and a half.
- 3x15 pulley down broad Grip I'm looking for a minute.

biceps:

- Pulldowns with a tight grip and biceps stripping 3 from a sequence of 6 + 6 + 6. I'm getting a minute and a half.
- Curl the three-by-ten cable. I'm looking for a minute.
- 3x10 arm carl machine I'm looking for a minute.
- -Card ranked sixth

-WORKOUT 06

MONDAY'

- Exercise your chest and triceps.

Chest:

- 3 sets of 12 chest presses with a broad grip. Obtain a minute.
- 4 sets of 6 chest presses with a tight grip, including a final repeat with 5 seconds rest. I'm looking for a minute.

- Crosses to the wires in three groups of twelve. Obtain a minute.

Triceps:

- Triceps cables 3x12 great reverse Grip I'm looking for a minute.
- Triceps cables 3x12 with ropes strong Grip I'm looking for a minute.

WEDNESDAY'

Workout for the Shoulders and Legs

Shoulders:

- 3 sets of 12 shoulder presses I'm looking for a minute.
- Raise the 3x10 cables in the front. I'm looking for a minute.

legs:

- Leg press 4x6. I'm looking for a minute.
- 3x6 Leg Extension I'm looking for a minute.
- 3x6 Leg Curls I'm looking for a minute.
- 3x8 calf sitting I'm looking for a minute.

FRIDAY'

- Training and biceps latissimusdorsi.
- Backbone:
- Lat Machine Jack Large Pyramid 4 sets of 15-10-7-4 repetitions. I am retrieving a minute.
- Pulley down, firm Grip, 4 sets of 15-10-7-4 repetitions, 1-minute rest.

biceps:

- 3 sets of 10 pulldowns with a tight grip and a handle on the biceps. Obtain a minute.
- Curl the three-by-twelve cable. I'm looking for a minute.
- 3x12 arm carl machine I'm looking for a minute.
- CARD is ranked 7th.

-WORKOUT 07

MONDAY'

- Exercise your chest and triceps.

Chest:

- 4 to 10-8-6-4 repetitions of the pyramid chest press (the load goes up). I'm looking for a minute.
- 3 sets of 10 dip machines Obtain a minute.
- Butterfly machine with three sets of ten. Obtain a minute.

Triceps:

- Triceps cables (rail) 3x10 wide Grip I'm looking for a minute.
- 3x10 triceps to grip cable reversal I'm looking for a minute.

WEDNESDAY'

- Workout for the Shoulders and Legs

Shoulders:

- 4 x 10-8-6-4 repetitions of the shoulder press pyramid (the load goes up). I'm looking for a minute.
- Raise the front three-by-twelve cables. I'm looking for a minute.

legs:

- 3x6 + 6 + 6 leg extension stripping I'm getting a minute and a half.
- Leg press 3x12. I'm looking for a minute.
- Stripping Leg Curls 3x6 + 6 + 6, I'm getting a minute and a half.
- 1xmax repetitions of calf standing.

FRIDAY'

- Training and biceps latissimusdorsi.

backbone:

- 4x6 repetitions of the Lat Machine wide grip pyramid. I'm looking for a minute.
- 4 × 6 repetitions with a broad grip on a pulley. I'm looking for a minute.

biceps:

- Pulldowns with a tight grip and a handle biceps 3 pyramidal series 3-6-9-12 (weight decreases) repetitions I'm looking for a minute.
- Curl the wire stripping 3 times in row 6 + 6 + 6. I'm getting a minute and a half.
    - CARD is ranked # 8 in the world.

-WORKOUT 08

MONDAY'

- Exercise your chest and triceps.

Chest:

- 4 6-8-12-15 repetitions of the pyramid chest press (the weight goes down). I'm looking for a minute.
- 3 sets of 10 dip machines Obtain a minute.
- Butterfly machine with three sets of ten. Obtain a minute.

Triceps:

- Triceppulldowns with a broad 3x8 grip I'm looking for a minute.
- Triceps to cable reverse grasp 3x8 I'm looking for a minute.

WEDNESDAY'

- Workout for the Shoulders and Legs

Shoulders:

- 3x8 shoulder press I'm looking for a minute.
- Raise the 3x8 wires in front of you. I'm looking for a minute.

legs:

- 4 to 3-6-9-12 reps on the leg press (the load goes down). I'm looking for a minute.
- 3x10 + 10 + 10 leg extension stripping Two minutes are being retrieved.
- 3 sets of 12 leg curls I'm looking for a minute.
- 3x15 calf sitting I'm looking for a minute.

FRIDAY'

- Training and biceps latissimusdorsi.

backbone:

- 3x8 repetitions of the Lat Machine wide grip pyramid. I'm looking for a minute.

biceps:

- The 4x8 cable should be curled. I'm looking for a minute.
- 3x10 arm carl machine I'm looking for a minute.
    - CARD is ranked 9th.

-WORKOUT 09

MONDAY'

- Exercise your chest and triceps.

Chest:

- 4x6 chest press I'm looking for a minute.
- 3 sets of 6 dip machines I'm looking for a minute.
- 3 sets of 6 butterfly machines In series 6 + 6 + 6, the last stripping was performed. I'm looking for a minute.

Triceps:

- 3x8 parallel triceps (with guided weight). I'm looking for a minute.
- 3x8 triceps strings I'm looking for a minute.

WEDNESDAY'

Legs exercise.

legs:

- 4-8-12-14 repetitions of press 4 from 4-8-12-14 repetitions of press 4 from 4-8-12-14 repeat (the weight goes down). I'm looking for a minute.
- 3x15 Leg Extensions I'm looking for a minute.
- Stripping Leg Curls 3x10 + 10 + 10 Two minutes are being retrieved.
- 3x15 calf sitting I'm looking for a minute.
- 1 x maximum calf standing

FRIDAY'

- Workout for the lats, biceps, and shoulders.

Shoulders:

- 3 sets of 10 shoulder presses I'm looking for a minute.
- Raise the 3x10 cables in the front. I'm looking for a minute.

backbone:

- 3x10 repetitions of a lat machine with a small pyramidal socket. I'm looking for a minute.
- 3x10 reps with a broad grip on a pulley. I'm looking for a minute.
- 3x10 repetitions of the Lat Machine broad grip pyramid. I'm looking for a minute.

biceps:

- Curl the three-by-six cable. I'm looking for a minute.
- 3x10 arm carl machine I'm looking for a minute.
- CARD is ranked #10 in the world.

MONDAY'

Exercise your chest and triceps.

Chest:

- 3 sets of 6 + 6 + 6 reps on the stripping chest press. I'm getting a minute and a half.
- I am stripping three sets of six, six, and six. I'm getting a minute and a half.
- Crosses to the wires in three groups of fifteen. Obtain a minute.

Triceps:

- Stripping socket for triceps cables (rail) 3x6 + 6 + 6. I'm getting a minute and a half.
- Triceps ropes to 3x12 ropes I'm looking for a minute.

WEDNESDAY'

Legs exercise.

legs:

- Strip 4x10 + 10 + 10 times. I'm getting a minute and a half.
- 3x15 Leg Extensions I'm looking for a minute.
- 3 sets of 15 leg curls I'm looking for a minute.
- 3x10 calf sitting I'm looking for a minute.
- 3x30 calf standing, I'm looking for a minute.

FRIDAY'

- Workout for the lats, biceps, and shoulders.

Shoulders:

- Stripping shoulder press 3x6 + 6 + 6, I'm getting a minute and a half.
- 3x10 + 10 + 10 cable stripping on the sides. I'm getting a minute and a half.

backbone:

- 3x8 repetitions of the Lat Machine wide grip pyramid. I'm looking for a minute.
- 6 + 6 + 6 repetitions of low grip narrow stripping using a pulley. I'm getting a minute and a half.

biceps:

- Strip the wires 3x6 + 6 + 6 curling. I'm getting a minute and a half.

-WORKOUT 11

Heating:

- Run for 5 minutes.
- Five minutes on the bike.
- stretching

Abdomen:

- 3 sets of 20 crunches. Obtain a minute.

lumbar:

- 2 sets of 15 reverse crunches per minute Recovery

Chest:

- Bench press with a barbell: 3 sets of 15 reps per minute Recovery

backbone:

- Pull-lat-machine: 3 sets of 15 repetitions per minute Recovery
- 2 sets of 15 latpulldowns per minute Recovery

Shoulders:

- Dumbbell push-ups: 3 sets of 15 per minute Recovery

biceps:

- Barbell curls: 3 sets of 15 with a minute rest in between.

Triceps:

- 3 sets of 12 cable pushdowns I'm looking for a minute.

legs:

- Press: 3 sets of 15 reps with a minute rest in between.

- Leg Curls: 3 sets of 15 with a minute rest in between.
- stretching

-WORKOUT 12

Heating:

Run for 5 minutes.
Five minutes on the bike.
stretching

Abdomen:

- 3 sets of 20 crunches. Obtain a minute.

Chest:

- Bench press with a barbell: 3 sets of 10 reps per minute Recovery
- Crosses to the cables: two sets of twelve. Obtain a minute.

backbone:

- Pull-lat-machine: 2 sets of 12 repetitions per minute Recovery
- Pulley: 2 sets of 12 repetitions per minute Recovery

Shoulders:

- 3 sets of 12 reps per minute with a pushed-up barbell Recovery

biceps:

- 2 sets of 12 dumbbell curls. Obtain a minute.

Triceps:

- Push down to the cables: two sets of twelve. Obtain a minute.

legs:

- Leg press: 2series (12 reps). Recover from a minute's worth of work.
- 2 sets of 12 leg curls. Obtain a minute.
- 2 sets of 12 deadlifts Obtain a minute.
- stretching

-WORKOUT 13

Heating:

- Run for 5 minutes.
- Five minutes on the bike.
- stretching

Abdomen:

- 3 times maximum crunch, I'm looking for a minute.

lumbar:

- 3 sets of 15 in a minute for reverse crunch recovery

Chest:

- 3 sets of 15 chest presses per minute Recovery

backbone:

- Pull-lat-machine: 3 sets of 15 repetitions per minute Recovery

Shoulders:

- Shoulder press: 3 sets of 15 reps per minute

biceps:

- Curl cables: 3 sets of 15 reps with a minute rest.

Triceps:

- Push down to the cables: three sets of twelve. I'm looking for a minute.

legs:

- Press: 3 sets of 15 reps with a minute rest in between.
- Leg Curls: 3 sets of 15 with a minute rest in between.
- stretching

Heating:

- Run for 5 minutes.
- Five minutes on the bike.
- stretching

Abdomen:

- 3 times maximum crunch, I'm looking for a minute.

lumbar:

- 3 sets of 10 per minute for reverse crunch recovery

Chest:

- 3 sets of 10 chest presses per minute Recovery

backbone:

- Pull-lat-machine: 3 sets of 10 reps per minute

Shoulders:

- Shoulder press: three sets of ten reps per minute Recovery

biceps:

- Curl cables come in three groups of ten. I'm looking for a minute.

Triceps:

- Push down to the cables in three sets of ten. I'm looking for a minute.

legs:

- 3 sets of 12 leg extensions. Obtain a minute.
- stretching

WORKOUT 15

MONDAY'

Heating.

backbone:

- 3 sets of 10 pulleys. Obtain a minute.
- Pull-lat-machine: three sets of ten. Obtain a minute.

Triceps:

- 3 sets of 8 French presses with a barbell I'm regaining a minute.

- There are two sets of ten ropes that connect to the wires. Obtain a minute.
- Abdominal, for example.

WEDNESDAY'

- Heating.

Shoulders:

- 3 sets of 12 shoulder presses. Obtain a minute.
- 2 sets of 10 face pull with a barbell. Obtain a minute.
- 2 sets of 12 dumbbell side openings. Obtain a minute.

legs:

- Leg extensions: three sets of ten. Obtain a minute.
- Leg curls: three sets of ten. Obtain a minute.
- Step calves: 1 x max.
- Abdominal, for example.

FRIDAY'

- Heating.

Chest:

- Chest Machine: three sets of ten. Obtain a minute.
- 2 sets of 8 on the Piana bench with dumbbells. I'm regaining a minute.

- 2 sets of 10 on the incline bench with a barbell. I'm regaining a minute.
- Crosses to the cables: two sets of twelve. Obtain a minute.

biceps:

- Curl the Cables: three sets of ten. Obtain a minute.
- 2 sets of 10 dumbbell curl hammer handle. Obtain a minute.
- 2 sets of 10 barbell curls. Obtain a minute.
- Abdominal, for example.

-WORKOUT 16

MONDAY'

Heating.

backbone:

- 4 sets of 6 pull-lat-machines I'm getting a minute and a half.
- 3 sets of 8 pulleys I'm regaining a minute.

Triceps:

- 4 sets of 6 French presses with a barbell I'm getting a minute and a half.
- 3 sets of 8 ropes to the cables I'm regaining a minute.

- Abdominal, for example.

WEDNESDAY'

Shoulders:

- 4 sets of 6 shoulder presses I'm getting a minute and a half.
- 2 sets of 8 face pull with a barbell; I'm regaining a minute.
- 3 sets of 10 dumbbell side openings. Obtain a minute.

legs:

- 4 sets of 6 leg extensions I'm getting a minute and a half.
- 3 sets of 8 leg curls I'm regaining a minute.
- Step calves: 1 x max.

FRIDAY'

- Heating.

Chest:

- 4 sets of 6 chest machines I'm getting a minute and a half.
- 3 sets of 8 incline barbell bench. I'm regaining a minute.

- Crosses to the cables: three groups of twelve. I'm looking for a minute.

biceps:

- Curl the cables in four sets of six. I'm getting a minute and a half.
- 3 sets of 8 dumbbell curl hammer handle I'm regaining a minute.
- Abdominal, for example.

-WORKOUT 17

MONDAY'

- Heating.

backbone:

- Pulley: 3 sets of 15 reps with a minute rest.
- Pull-lat-machine: 3 sets of 15 reps with a minute rest in between.

Triceps:

- Push down to the cables: 3 sets of 15 reps with a minute rest.
- 2 sets of 15 a minute recovery from the rope to the cables.
- Abdominal, for example.

WEDNESDAY'

- Heating.

Shoulders:

- Shoulder press: 3 sets of 15 reps with a minute rest in between.
- Raise the front cables by 3x15. I'm looking for a minute.

legs:

- Leg Extensions: 3 sets of 15 with a minute rest in between.
- Leg curls: 3 sets of 15 with a minute rest in between.
- 3x15 calf seated, I'm looking for a minute.
- Abdominal, for example.

FRIDAY'

- Heating.

Chest:

- Chest Machine: 3 sets of 15 reps with a minute rest in between.
- Dip parallel to the machine: 3 sets of 15 with a minute rest in between.

- Crosses to the cables: 3 sets of 15 with a minute rest in between.

biceps:

- Curl the Cables: 3 sets of 15 reps with a minute rest.
- 3 sets of 15 curl scott to cables Obtain a minute.
- Abdominal, for example.

-WORKOUT 18

- MONDAY'
- Heating.

backbone:

- Pull-lat-machine broad grip: 3 sets of 15 reps with a minute rest.
- Pulley: 3 sets of 15 reps with a minute rest.
- Close pull-lat-machine socket: 3 sets of 15 per minute recovery.

Triceps:

- Push down to the cables: 3 sets of 15 reps with a minute rest.
- Rope to cables: 3 sets of 15 reps with a minute rest.
- Abdominal, for example.

WEDNESDAY'

- Heating.

legs:

- 3 sets of 10 presses. Obtain a minute.
- Leg Extensions: 3 sets of 15 with a minute rest in between.
- Leg curls: 3 sets of 15 with a minute rest in between.
- 3x15 calf seated, I'm looking for a minute.
- 1 x maximum calf standing
- Abdominal, for example.

FRIDAY'

- Heating.

Chest:

- Chest wide grip machine: 2 sets of 15 reps with a minute rest.
- Chest Machine socket tight: 2 sets of 15 reps with a minute rest.
- Crosses to the cables: 2 sets of 15 with a minute rest in between.

biceps:

- Curl with hammer grip dumbbells: 3 sets of 15 reps with a minute rest.
- Curl scott to cables: 3 sets of 15 reps with a minute rest.
- Abdominal, for example.

-WORKOUT 19

- TUESDAY'

Heating:

- 5 minutes of gentle running
- Five minutes on the bike.

abs:

- 3x10 crunch I'm looking for a minute.

Chest:

- Bench 3x12 in size. I'm looking for a minute.
- 30'3x12 dumbbell incline bench presses one minute of rest

biceps:

- 3x12 dumbbell curls standing. I'm looking for a minute.

Triceps:

- 3x12 French press I'm looking for a minute.

THURSDAY'

Heating:

- 5 minutes of gentle running
- Five minutes on the bike.

Shoulders:

- 3 sets of 12 shoulder presses I'm looking for a minute.

backbone:

- 3x12 squats on the lat machine I'm looking for a minute.

legs:

- 3x12 print. I'm looking for a minute.
- I am retrieving a minute with 3x12 leg curls.
- Calf standing number one x maximum repetitions

-WORKOUT 20

TUESDAY'

Heating:

- 5 minutes of gentle running
- Five minutes on the bike.
- abs:
- 4x8 crunch I'm looking for a minute.

Chest:

- Presses 4x6 on a flat bench. I'm getting a minute and a half.
- Bench presses on an incline of 30'3x8 using dumbbells. one minute of rest
- The 2x10 cable is crossed. I'm looking for a minute.

biceps:

- 4x6 dumbbell curls standing I'm getting a minute and a half.

Triceps:

- 4x6 French press I'm getting a minute and a half.

THURSDAY'

Heating:

- 5 minutes of gentle running
- Five minutes on the bike.

Shoulders:

- 4x6 shoulder press I'm getting a minute and a half.
- Raise the front 2x10 times. I'm looking for a minute.

backbone:

- 4x6 forward lat machine I'm getting a minute and a half.
- Below a 2x10 sprocket, a sprocket I'm looking for a minute.

legs:

- 4x6 print. I'm getting a minute and a half.
- 3 sets of 10 leg curls I'm looking for a minute.
- 2x10 calf sitting I'm looking for a minute.

-WORKOUT 21

- Heating.
- 5 minutes of gentle running to the mat
- Five minutes on the bike.

Abdomen:

- 3 x15 crunch 45 seconds of rest

lumbar:

- 3x15 reverse crunch 45 seconds of rest

Chest:

- 1x15 chest press You go on to the next exercise without taking a break.

Shoulders:

- 1x15 face pulls using a barbell. You go on to the next exercise without taking a break.
- 1x15 military press with barbell You go on to the next exercise without taking a break.
- 1x15 side openings with dumbbells You go on to the next exercise without taking a break.

backbone:

- 1x15 lat-machine reverse Grip You go on to the next exercise without taking a break.
- All of this was done three times.

-WORKOUT 22

- Heating.

- 5 minutes of gentle running to the mat

- Five minutes on the bike.

Abdomen:

- 1x15 sit-ups You go on to the next exercise without stopping, and so on.

Chest:

- 1 x15 bench press

backbone:

- 1x15 Lat Machine Reverse

Shoulders:

- 1x15 military press with dumbbells or machine

legs:

- 1x15 Leg Extending
- 1x15 Leg Curls
- 1x15 Leg Press

biceps:

- 1x15 Standing Dumbbell Curl

Triceps:

- 1x15 Triceps to cable with a rope

calves:

- 1x15 calf machine
- The whole thing is repeated three times.

-WORKOUT 23

- Heating.
- 5 minutes of gentle running to the mat
- Five minutes on the bike.

Abdomen:

- 3x15 crunch, 1-minute rest

Chest:

- 3x15 on the chest machine, 1-minute rest.

backbone:

- Next: 3x15 on the lat machine, followed by a minute of rest.

Shoulders:

- 3x15 military press with dumbbells or machine, 1-minute rest.

legs:

- Leg extension: 3x15, 1 minute rest.
- Leg curls: 3x15, 1-minute rest.
- Leg press: 3x15, 1-minute rest.

biceps:

- 3x15 Standing Dumbbell Curls, 1-minute rest.

Triceps:

- Triceps cables: 3x15, 1-minute rest.

calves:

- 3x15 on the calf machine, 1-minute rest.
- -card 24

-WORKOUT 24

-MONDAY':

- Heating.

Chest:

- 4 sets of 10 reps of flat bench presses I'm looking for a minute.
- Bench incline to 45 degrees: 3 sets of 10 repetitions I'm looking for a minute.

- Crosses to the cables or 45-degree incline bench: 2 sets of 12. Obtain a minute.

Shoulders:

- 4x10 military press I'm looking for a minute.
- 3x10 side risers are standing; I'm looking for a minute.

Triceps:

- 3 x8 parallel bodyweight (or machine assistance) for triceps. I'm looking for a minute.
- 3 x10 French press with a barbell I'm looking for a minute.

Abdomen:

- 3 sets of 20 crunches per minute Recovery

etc.

-WEDNESDAY':

- Heating.

legs:

- 2x12 Leg Extensions I'm looking for a minute. (light)
- 4x12 squats I'm looking for a minute.
- 3 sets of 12 lunges I'm looking for a minute.
- Restore a minute by cutting to 3x12.

- 1x max repetitions of calves calf standing

-FRIDAY':

- Heating.

backbone:

- Free-body tractions
- 4x10 squats on the lat machine I'm looking for a minute.

biceps:

- 4x10 barbell curls I'm looking for a minute.
- 3 x 10 curl scott, I'm looking for a minute.

Abdomen:

- 3 sets of 20 crunches per minute Recovery
- Isometric abdominal exercise.
- CARD NO. 25
- MONDAY'S THEME: HEATING. Crunches: 3 sets of 10 per minute Recovery, etc.

-WORKOUT 25

-MONDAY':

- Heating.

Chest:

- 4x6 flat bench presses I'm getting a minute and a half.
- 3x8 incline bench presses with dumbbells at 45 degrees: 3x8 recovery per minute
- Dumbbell crosses on the incline bench at 45 degrees: 2x10. 45 seconds were added.

Triceps:

- 4x6 parallel for triceps, I'm getting a minute and a half.
- 3x8 French Press I'm looking for a minute.
- 3x10 cables I'm looking for a minute.

Abdomen:

- 3 sets of 15 crunches per minute Recovery
- etc.

-WEDNESDAY':

- Heating.

legs:

- 4x6 squats I'm getting a minute and a half.
- 3x8 lunges I'm looking for a minute.
- 2x10 leg extensions I'm looking for a minute.
- 4x6 deadlift I'm getting a minute and a half.

- 2x10 leg curls I'm looking for a minute.
- 3x10 seated calf I'm looking for a minute.

-FRIDAY':

- Heating.

Shoulders:

- 4x6 military press with a barbell I'm getting a minute and a half.
- Raise fronts super series 3x10 with lateral raises. I'm getting a minute and a half.
- backbone:
- 4x6 lat machine I'm getting a minute and a half.
- 3x10 rower with handlebar I'm looking for a minute.

biceps:

- curlscott: 3x6. Recupero a minute and a half
- Dumbbells with a grip: 3x10. Hammer: 3x10. I'm looking for a minute.
- CARD NO. 26

-WORKOUT 26

-MONDAY':

- Heating.

Abdomen:

- 3 sets of 10 crunches per minute Recovery
- etc.

Chest:

- 4x6 incline bench presses I'm getting a minute and a half.
- 3x6 Piana Bench Presses I'm getting a minute and a half.
- 3x10 cross-overs to the cables I'm looking for a minute.

Shoulders:

- 4x6 military press with dumbbells I'm getting a minute and a half.
- 3x6 raised side by sitting; I'm getting a minute and a half.

Triceps:

- 4x6 cable pushdown I'm getting a minute and a half.
- 3x6 with handlebars behind your head. I'm getting a minute and a half.

-WEDNESDAY':

- Heating.

legs:

- 3x10 leg extensions I'm looking for a minute.
- 4x6 squats I'm getting a minute and a half.
- 3x6 lunges, 1 minute and a half rest.
- 3x6 deadlift I'm getting a minute and a half.
- 3x6 Leg Curls. Rest a minute and a half.
- Calves calf standing: 1 x max repetitions. 1-minute retrieval
- 3x10 calves calf sitting I'm looking for a minute.

-FRIDAY':

- Heating.

backbone:

- 4x6 rower barbell I'm getting a minute and a half.
- 3x6 on the lat machine with a thin grip. Rest for a minute and a half.
- 3x6 low pulley I'm getting a minute and a half.

biceps:

- 4x6 standing dumbbells I'm getting a minute and a half.
- 3x6 curl scott, I'm getting a minute and a half.
- abdominal

- CARD 27

-WORKOUT 27

-MONDAY':

- Heating.

Chest:

- 4 sets of 14-10-7-4 pyramid flat bench presses. Taking a minute and a half...
- 3x6 flat bench presses with incline dumbbell bench. I'm getting a minute and a half.
- 3x10 cross-overs to the cables I'm looking for a minute.

Triceps:

- 4x6 parallel for triceps, I'm getting a minute and a half.
- 3x6 French Press I'm getting a minute and a half.
- 3x10 with ropes I'm looking for a minute.

-WEDNESDAY':

- Heating.

legs:

- 5 sets of 14-11-9-6-3 squats I'm getting a minute and a half.

- 3x10 leg extensions I'm looking for a minute.
- 3x10 walking lunges I'm looking for a minute.
- 3x10 deadlifts I'm looking for a minute.
- 3x10 leg curls I'm looking for a minute.
- 3x8 calf sitting I'm looking for a minute.

-FRIDAY':

- Heating.

backbone:

- 5 sets of 14-11-9-6-3 on the wide grip lat machine. I'm getting a minute and a half.
- 3x6 rower barbell I'm getting a minute and a half.

Shoulders:

- 5 sets of 14-11-9-6-3 dumbbell military press I'm getting a minute and a half.
- 3x6 front increases I'm getting a minute and a half.

biceps:

- 4x8 standing barbell I'm looking for a minute.
- 3x8 curl scott, I'm looking for a minute.
- Abs.
- CARD NO. 28

-MONDAY':

Chest:

- Flat bench presses: 4 sets of 6 + 6 + 6 (weight goes down without rest). Rest a minute and a half.
- Stripping 3 sets of 6 + 6 + 6 incline bench presses with dumbbells, I'm getting a minute and a half.
- Standing crosses to the cables: 2 x10. 45 seconds of rest

Shoulders:

- Stripping 4 sets of 6 + 6 + 6 military press with dumbbells, I'm getting a minute and a half.

Triceps:

- Push the machine down: 3 sets of 8 + 6 + 6. I'm getting a minute and a half.
- Dumbbell: 3x10 in stripping Series 10 + 6 + 6.
- abdominal

-WEDNESDAY':

legs:

- 3x10 leg extensions I'm looking for a minute.

- Squat: 3 sets of 8 + 6 + 6 squats I'm getting a minute and a half.
- 3 sets of 12 lunges I'm looking for a minute.
- When the last is stripped 10 + 8 + 8, cut to 3x10. I'm looking for a minute.
- 3 sets of 10 leg curls I'm looking for a minute.

-FRIDAY':

backbone:

- Stripping 4 sets of 6 + 6 + 6 + 6 on the lat machine. I'm getting a minute and a half.
- Rower barbell: 3x10, with the final rep consisting of stripping 10 + 8 + 8. I'm looking for a minute.

biceps:

- Standing dumbbell stripping: 4 sets of 6 + 6 + 6. Rest a minute and a half.
- 3x8 curl scott, I'm looking for a minute.
- Abs.
- CARD NO. 29

-WORKOUT 29

- -MONDAY'

Chest:

- 4 sets of 15-11-7-3 repetitions on the bench press pyramid.

backbone:

- 4 pyramidal series of 15-11-7-3 repetitions on the rower with a barbell.
- They are now training lats and chest with three super series. 3 supersets are completed with 8 repetitions of:
- Dumbbells on an incline bench
- -laundry machine
- Traverses cables
- -Pull-ups with a dumbbell
- These workouts are done without a break. Following completing a superset, the second after the break begins. The recuperation time varies from 2 to 3 minutes.

Abdomen:

- 3 sets of 20 crunches per minute Recovery

lumbar:

- 3 sets of 15 reverse crunch 40 seconds of rest

-WEDNESDAY'

legs:

- FTL barbell deadlift 4 pyramidal series 14-11-8-5 reps
- 4 pyramidal series of inclined presses 14-11-8-5 repetitions
- Now do several supersets of exercises. 3 are 8-rep supersets of:
- -extension of the legs
- -Lunges with dumbbells
- -leg curling
- The recuperation time varies from 2 to 3 minutes.

ON FRIDAY:

- 14-11-8-5 repetitions military press 4 pyramidal series
- 4 pyramidal sets of 14-11-8-5 repetitions on the face pull
- Now do several supersets of exercises. 3 are 8-rep supersets of:
- -Barbell Curl (wide opening hands)
- -Cables Triceps
- -Jack hammer with a curl Dumbbell

Abdomen:

- 3 sets of 20 crunches. Obtain a minute.

lumbar:

- 3 sets of 15 reverse crunch 40 seconds of rest.
- -card 30

- -MONDAY'

abs:

- 3x30 crunch 45 seconds of rest
- Chest:
- 6 x 4 repetitions on the flat bench (weight around 85 percent of the ceiling). I'm looking for a minute.
- 6x4 parallel to the incline I'm looking for a minute.
- The 3x10 cable is crossed. I'm looking for a minute.
- Triceps
- 6x4 cables I'm looking for a minute.

-WEDNESDAY'

Abdomen:

- Performed under isometric tension with his toes and elbows elevated. 1 minute of isometric tension

backbone:

- 6x4 rower barbell I'm looking for a minute.
- Forward Lat Machine 6x4 I'm looking for a minute.

biceps:

- 6x4 barbell curls I'm looking for a minute.
- 6x4 curl scott, I'm looking for a minute.

-FRIDAY'

- abs:
- 3x30 crunch 45 seconds of rest

Shoulders:

- 6x4 military press dumbbells I'm looking for a minute.
- 3x10 side risers one minute of rest

legs:

- Squats with a barbell for a 6x4 free body. I'm looking for a minute.
- I completed 6x4 deadlifts. I'm looking for a minute.
- CARD 31 -

-WORKOUT 31

-MONDAY'

Chest:

- 5 sets of 12-10-8-6-3 reps on the flat bench press. A minute/minute and a half are being retrieved.

- 30'3 sets of 8 incline bench presses I'm regaining a minute.
- Crosses on the bench (30'3 sets of 12) Obtain a minute.

Shoulders:

- 12-10-8-6-3 repetitions of the military press 5 series A minute/minute and a half is being retrieved.
- 3 sets of 12 side risers. Obtain a minute.

Triceps:

- 12-10-8-6-3 5 sets of repetitions on an incline bench, retrieving a minute/minute and a half.
- Triceps cables (push-down cables) come in three sets of twelve. Obtain a minute.

-WEDNESDAY'

legs:

- Leg extension three times with a ten-minute rest in between.
- 5 sets of 12-10-8-6-3 repetitions squat A minute/minute and a half is being retrieved.
- 3 sets of 10 lunges I'm looking for a minute.
- 3x10 deadlifts with a minute rest.
- 3x10 calves calf sitting I'm looking for a minute.

-FRIDAY'

backbone:

- 5 sets of 12-10-8-6-3 reps on the lat machine. A minute/minute and a half are being retrieved.
- Pull down three sets of ten. Obtain a minute.
- 3 sets of 10 rows with a dumbbell. Obtain a minute.

biceps:

- Curl the barbell 5 times for 5 sets of 12-10-8-6-3 reps. A minute/minute and a half are being retrieved.
- 3 sets of 12 curl scott curl scott curl scott curl scott curl s Obtain a minute.
- -card 32

-WORKOUT 32

-MONDAY'

Chest:

- Bench presses 1x10 on the flat. I'm looking for a minute.
- 30'1x10'Recupero a minute in line bench presses 30'1x10'Recupero a minute'Recupero a minute'Recuper
- 30 '1x10 bench crosses I'm looking for a minute.

- The preceding three exercises are performed three times. *

Shoulders:

- 1x10 repetitions of military press I'm looking for a minute.
- 1x10 side risers I'm looking for a minute.
- The preceding two exercises are performed three times. *

Triceps:

- 1x10 repetitions of the French press on an incline bench. I'm looking for a minute.
- 1x10 triceps cables (push-down cables) I'm looking for a minute.
- The preceding two exercises are performed three times. *

-WEDNESDAY'

legs:

- 1 × 10 Leg Extensions I'm looking for a minute.
- 1x10 repetitions of squats I'm looking for a minute.
- 1x10 Lunges I'm looking for a minute.
- 1x10 deadlifts with a minute rest.
- 1x10 calves calf sitting I'm looking for a minute.

- The preceding five exercises are performed three times. *

-FRIDAY'

backbone:

- 1x10 reps on the lat machine. I'm looking for a minute.
- Below a 1x10 sprocket, a sprocket I'm looking for a minute.
- 1x10 rowing with a barbell. I'm looking for a minute.
- The three exercises are performed three times. *

biceps:

- 1x10 curl standing I'm looking for a minute.
- 1x10 curl scott, I'm looking for a minute.
- The preceding two exercises are performed three times. *
- CARD NO. 33

-WORKOUT 33

-MONDAY'

Chest:

- To workout, do four Super 8 reps:
- The bench press is a kind of exercise that involves the use of

- Attempts to cross the wires.
- Bench presses on an incline.
- There is no rest time between exercises. After the superset, there is a period of recovery.
- I'm taking a two-minute break.

Shoulders:

- 3 supersets of 8 repetitions for each exercise:
- the military press
- The front rises.
- Risers on the sides.
- There is no rest time between exercises. After the superset, there is a period of recovery.
- I'm taking a two-minute break.

Triceps:

- Three supersets of eight repetitions each exercise:
- Parallel triceps.
- The French Press.
- Push your way down to the wires.
- There is no rest time between exercises. After the superset, there is a period of recovery.
- I'm taking a two-minute break.

-WEDNESDAY'

legs:

- Quadriceps 4 Super 8 repetitions to do:
- Squat.
- Leg Extending.
- Lunges.
- There is no rest time between exercises. Recovery takes place at the
- the end of the superset
- I'm taking a two-minute break.
- To exercise, do 3 super 8 repetitions on the femur:
- Deadlifts.
- Curl your legs.
- There is no rest time between exercises. After the superset, there is a period of recovery. *
- I'm taking a two-minute break.
- 2 supersets of 10 repetitions on the calves:
- Standing calf
- The calf is seated.
- There is no rest time between exercises. After the superset, there is a period of recovery. *
- I'm getting a minute and a half.

-FRIDAY'

backbone:

- To workout, do four Super 8 reps:
- Latpulldowns with a wide grip.
- rowing while hunched over
- Narrow Grip on the lat machine.
- There is no rest time between exercises. After the superset, there is a period of recovery. *
- I'm taking a two-minute break.

biceps:

- To workout, do three Super 8 reps:
- Curl with a barbell
- Scott, curl
- Curl the handle of a standing hammer.
- There is no rest time between exercises. After the superset, there is a period of recovery. *
- I'm taking a two-minute break.
- Card No. 34

-WORKOUT 34

- 'MONDAY, WEDNESDAY, AND FRIDAY'
- Heating.
- stretching

Abdomen:

- 3 sets of 20 crunches. Obtain a minute.

lumbar:

- Prono extensions on the bench: 2 sets of 15 per minute, 1-minute rest.

Chest:

- Push-ups: 3 sets of 15 reps per minute. 1 minute of rest.

back:

- Bodyweight horizontal pull-ups: 3 sets of 15 per minute. Recovery

Shoulders:

- 3 sets of 15 push-ups per minute Recovery

biceps:

- Chin-ups: 3 sets of 15 with a minute rest in between.

Triceps:

- 3 sets of 12 incline push-ups. Obtain a minute.

legs:

- Leg Extension Chair: 3 sets of 15 reps with a minute rest in between.
- Squats: 3 sets of 15 with a minute rest in between.
- stretching
- -card 35

MONDAY'

- Heating.
- back:
- Wide push-ups: 3 sets of 15 with a minute rest in between.
- Bodyweight horizontal pull-ups: 3 sets of 15 with a minute rest in between.

Triceps:

- Push-ups with diamonds: 3 sets of 15 with a minute rest in between.
- Triceps using a chair: 3 sets of 15 with a minute rest in between.

Glutes:

- Donkey kicks: 3 sets of 15 with a minute rest in between.

abs:

- 3x15 reverse crunch I'm looking for a minute.
- 3x15 sitting twist Take a minute to recover.
- 3x30 heel touches I'm looking for a minute.

WEDNESDAY'

- Heating.

Shoulders:

- Pick push-ups: 3 sets of 15 with a minute rest in between.
- 3x15 Hindu push-ups I'm looking for a minute.

legs:

- Chair leg extension: 3 sets of 15 with a minute rest in between.
- Sumo Squats: 3 sets of 15 with a minute rest in between.
- 3 sets of 15 walking lunges I'm looking for a minute.
- 3x30 calf standing, I'm looking for a minute.

FRIDAY'

- Heating.

Chest:

- Push up handles: 3 sets of 15 reps with a minute rest.
- Dip the parallel bars (chairs): 3 sets of 15 reps with a minute rest.
- Large push-ups: 3 sets of 15 with a minute rest.

Glutes:

- Bridges: 3 sets of 15 with a minute rest in between.

abs:

- 3x30 plank arm raises I'm looking for a minute.
- 3x30 seconds side plank without a recovery side
- -Card 36

-WORKOUT 36

- 'MONDAY, WEDNESDAY, AND FRIDAY'
- 3x10 wide push up I'm looking for a minute.
- 3x10 push-ups with your legs up. I'm looking for a minute.
- 3x10 squats I'm looking for a minute.
- 3x10 should be pulled up. I'm looking for a minute.
- 3x50-second planks I'm looking for a minute.
- 3x40 seconds of side plank. I'm looking for a minute.
- Card No. 37

-WORKOUT 37

MONDAY'

Chest:

- Recovery two minutes. 4 x12 push-ups with rest-pause technique (The rest-pause technique consists of completing as many repeats as possible. You rest 10 seconds, start again, make all the repetitions you can, repeat after 10 seconds of rest till 10/12, etc.
- They are pushing up 3x8 and retrieving a minute.

biceps:

- Curl with bottles 3x12 for a minute.

abs:

- Crunch 3 times maximum while retrieving a minute.
- 3x40 seconds of side plank.

TUESDAY'

legs:

- Squat 4x12 with a two-minute break in between.
- I am retrieving a minute using a 3x12 leg extension chair.
- Sumo squats in three supersets of 12 repetitions each, followed by side lunges.
- Step 3x6 lunges, recovering a minute and a half.

THURSDAY'

Shoulders:

- Pick up pushups 4x12 using the rest-pause technique, recovering for two minutes.
- I am retrieving a minute using side risers made of bottles or elastic 3x12.
- I am retrieving a minute using elastic bottles or 3x12.

Triceps:

- 4x12 in parallel using the rest-pause technique, with a two-minute recovery period.
- Diamonds are pushing up 3x8 and retrieving a minute.

FRIDAY

back:

- 4x12 horizontal pull-ups with bodyweight retrieving a minute
- 3x10 pull-ups using the rest-pause technique, resting for two minutes.

limbs:

- 4x8 bodyweight deadlifts with a minute rest.
- 3x10 sumo squats, 1 minute rest.
- Calf standing 2xmax and retrieving a minute

- -Card 38

- MONDAY'

Chest:

- 3x maximum dip parallel.
- Push-ups 5x8x8x8x8x8x8x8x8x8x8x8x
- Push-ups with 4x8 grips. I am retrieving a minute.
- Push up wide three times, 15 times, and ten times. Rest for one minute.

back:

- 3x12 hyperextensions retrieving a minute
- I am retrieving a minute with a 3x8 pull-up reversal.
- Bodyweight horizontal pull-ups 3x8. I am retrieving a minute.
- I am retrieving a minute while doing a star plank 3xmax seconds.

abs:

- 3x30 heel taps, retrieving a minute
- I am retrieving a minute after 3x30 crunches.

WEDNESDAY'

legs:

- Squat leg 4x10 8 6 4 for a minute and a half.
- 3x20 side leg lifts 1-minute rest.
- 3x8 lunges, 1-minute rest.
- Chair leg extensions 3x12. I am retrieving a minute.
- Calf standing 4x15 for a minute.

FRIDAY'

- Shoulders:
- 4x8 burpees while retrieving a minute
- 3x10 Hindu push-ups retrieving a minute

biceps:

- I am obtaining a minute and a half by pulling up reverse grip 3x 8 6 4.
- Pseudo plank 2x max. 1-minute retrieval

Triceps:

- 3 x 8 6 4 retrieving a minute
- -card 39

-WORKOUT 39

MONDAY'

- Triceps and chest:
- I am retrieving a minute with 4x12-10-8-6 push-up grips.
- Push up wide 4x12-10-8-6 for a minute.
- I am retrieving a minute with a 4x10 dip parallel.
- Diamonds push up 3x10 for a minute.
- 4x10 incline push-ups retrieving a minute

WEDNESDAY'

- 4x12-10-8-6 wide-grip pull-ups in a minute.
- 4x12-10-8-6 horizontal pull up bodyweight retrieving a minute
- Pull up 4x12-10-8-6 and wait a minute.
- Pseudo plank 3x50 seconds while retrieving a minute

abs:

- 3x20 Bicycle crunches while retrieving a minute
- 3x max side plank hip lifts in a minute.

FRIDAY'

- Shoulders and legs:
- Chair leg extensions 4x12-10-8-6. I am retrieving a minute.

- Lunges 4x10, 1-minute rest.

- 3x30 calf standing, 1-minute retrieval

- 3x12 sumo squats, 1 minute rest.

- Pick and push up 4x12-10-8-6 for a minute.

- 4x10 elastic shoulder side retrieving a minute.

- 4x10 elastic shoulder front retrieving a minute.

- -card 40

-WORKOUT 40

TUESDAY'

- Chest:

- 4x6 push-ups, 2 minutes rest.

Shoulders:

- 3x6 Hindu push-ups with a two-minute rest.

back:

- 3x6 bodyweight horizontal pull-ups, 2 minutes rest.

- I am recovering for two minutes with a 3x6 pull-up bar.

Triceps:

- I am retrieving a minute and a half after a 3x8 dip between two seats.

biceps:

- I am retrieving a minute, and a half for doorframes rows 3x8.

THURSDAY'

legs:

- 4x6 sumo squats with a two-minute rest.
- 3x6 plank jump with a two-minute rest.
- Donkey kicks 3x6 and rests for two minutes.
- Fly 3x6 steps, then recover for two minutes.
- 4x6 walking lunges with a two-minute rest.
- Calf standing 3x15 for a minute and a half, retrieving for a minute and a half.
- -Card 41

-WORKOUT 41

MONDAY'

legs:

- Squat 5x5 on one leg, recovering for two and a half minutes.
- Fly 3x6 steps for a minute and a half.
- 3x6 lunges on the step for a minute and a half.
- Slow bodyweight deadlift 4x6 with a minute and a half recovery.

- 3x10 calf raises 1-minute rest.

Chest:

- Push-ups 5x5, resting for two and a half minutes.
- 4x6 push-ups on the floor, retrieving a minute and a half.

Triceps:

- 4x6 parallel to the triceps, 1 minute and 15 seconds.
- 4x6 diamond push-ups in a minute and a half.

FRIDAY'

Shoulders:

- 5x5 Hindu push-ups, resting two and a half minutes.
- 3x8 burpees, retrieving a minute and a half.

back:

- 4x6 wide-grip pull-ups in a minute and a half.
- I am retrieving a minute and a half with a push up wide grip 4x6.

biceps:

- 4x6 with chins firm Grip and a minute and a half recovery
- -card 42

-WORKOUT 42

- MONDAY'

Chest:

- Push-ups 4x8 for a minute and a half.
- 3x8 push-ups with legs on upwards, retrieving a minute and a half.

Shoulders:

- Pike push-ups 5x8 in a minute and a half.

back:

- 3x8 chin-ups in a minute and a half.

abs:

- Retrieving a minute after 3x10 crunches.
- I am retrieving a minute by doing 3x50-second planks.
- I am retrieving a minute with 3x40 second broadside planks.

WEDNESDAY'

legs:

- Squat 3x8 for a minute and a half.
- 3x8 lunges and a minute and a half of retrieval
- Retrieving a minute and a half. Leg Extension Chair 3x8.
- 3x10 calf raises followed by a minute and a half of retrieval.

Triceps:

- 3x8 diamond push-ups in a minute and a half.

biceps:

- Curl up 3x8 with elastic and retrieve for a minute and a half.

FRIDAY'

- Chest:
- Push-ups 4x8 for a minute and a half.
- 3x8 push-ups with legs on upwards, retrieving a minute and a half.

Shoulders:

- 5x8 Hindu push-ups in a minute and a half.

back:

- 3x8 pull-ups on the rear bar in a minute and a half.

abs:

- Retrieving a minute with 3x10 bicycle crunches.
- I am retrieving a minute by doing 3x50-second planks.
- I am retrieving a minute with 3x40 second broadside planks.
- -Card 43

-WORKOUT 43

TUESDAY'

Abdomen:

- Retrieving a minute with a Russian 3x10 twist.
- I am retrieving a minute by doing 3x50-second planks.
- I am retrieving a minute with 3x40 second broadside planks.

Chest:

- Push up 3x8-6-4 repetitions for a minute and a half.

biceps:

- 3x8-6-4 repetitions on the chin up, retrieving a minute and a half.

Triceps:

- Diamonds push up 3x8-6-4 repetitions, recovering 1 minute and 15 seconds.

legs:

- Step 3x8-6-4 repetitions of lunges, recovering a minute and a half.

THURSDAY'

Shoulders:

- 3x8-6-4 repetitions of Hindu push-ups in a minute and a half.

back:

- 3x8-6-4 repetitions of wide-grip pull-ups in a minute and a half.

legs:

- 3x8-6-4 squats in a minute and a half.

Abdomen:

- Retrieving a minute after 3x10 crunches.
- 3x10 leg raises, 1-minute rest.
- -card 44

-WORKOUT 44

- 'THURSDAY AND TUESDAY'

Chest:

- Push-ups pyramidal 7x12-10-8-6-10-12, two-minute rest.

back:

- Push up wide opening 7x12-10-8-6-10-12, two minutes rest.

legs:

- Squat pyramids 7x12-10-8-6-10-12, two minutes rest.
- CARD 45

-WORKOUT 45

MONDAY'

Chest:

- Push-ups 5 times (8-6-4-6-8), she is recovering for a minute and a half.

Back:

- 3x10 horizontal pull-ups with a one-minute rest

- Pull up pyramidal bar 5x 8-6-4-6-8 in 1 minute and 15 seconds.

WEDNESDAY'

- biceps:
- 5x 8-6-4-6-8 horizontal pull-ups in a minute and a half.

Triceps:

- 3x10 diamond push-ups retrieving a minute
- Dip between seats 5 times (8-6-4-6-8), recovering for a minute and a half.

FRIDAY'

Shoulders:

- 3 × 10 elastic raised side retrieving a minute
- Pike push up pyramidal 5x 8-6-4-6-8 in 1 minute and 15 seconds.

legs:

- I am retrieving a minute using a leg extension 3x10 chair.
- Squat pyramids 5x 8-6-4-6-8 in 1:45.
- -Card 46

MONDAY'

- Shoulders and lower back:

- 3x3 burpees with a minute rest.

- 3 sets of 3 Hindu push-ups with one-minute rest.

- I am recovering for two minutes after a 3x8 pull-up.

- I am retrieving a minute with a horizontal pull up bodyweight 3xmax.

- I am retrieving a minute with a 5xmax star plank.

TUESDAY'

legs:

- 1x20 Leg Extension Chair

- 3x10 bridges. 1-minute retrieval

- 3x15 sumo squats, 1 minute rest.

- Lunges on step 4x6 with a two-minute rest.

- 3x15 leg raises on the side, retrieving a minute.

Abdomen:

- Retrieving a minute with 3x20 heel taps.

- I am retrieving a minute with 3x20 bicycle crunches.

WEDNESDAY'

Chest:

- I am retrieving a minute while clapping push-ups three times.
- Push-ups three times maximum. I am retrieving a minute.
- Push up handles three times maximum, retrieving a minute.
- I am retrieving a minute after a 3xmax dip.
- 3x30 plank rotations with a minute recovery.

FRIDAY'

Arms:

- Bodyweight 4x8 horizontal pull-ups I'm looking for a minute.
- Pseudo plank 4x maximum. I'm looking for a minute.
- Dip on the chairs three times maximum. I'm looking for a minute.
- 3 sets of 10 push-ups I'm looking for a minute.
- Diamonds increase the maximum by 3x. I'm looking for a minute.
- -Card 47

-WORKOUT 47

MONDAY'

Chest:

- Push up handles that are 6x8 in size. 40 seconds of rest.
- 6x8 push-ups with legs up. 40 seconds of rest.
- Push up a really big 3x15 image. 40 seconds of rest.

Triceps:

- 6x8 incline pushes up 40 seconds of rest.
- Dip parallel for 6x8 triceps. 40 seconds of rest.

WEDNESDAY'

legs:

- 3 x 20 Leg Extension Chair I'm looking for a minute.
- 6x8 sumo squat 40 seconds of rest.
- Donkey scores a 6x8. 40 seconds of rest.
- 6x8 lunges 40 seconds of rest.

abs:

- 3x20 Bicycle crunches I'm looking for a minute.
- 3x maximum side plank hip raise. I'm looking for a minute.
- 3x15 oblique v ups I'm looking for a minute.

FRIDAY'

backbone:

- 6x8 pull-up bar 40 seconds of rest.
- 6x8 horizontal pull up bodyweight 40 seconds of rest.

Shoulders:

- 6x8 Hindu push-ups 40 seconds of rest.
- 6x8 burpees 40 seconds of rest.

biceps:

- Pseudo plank 3x maximum. I'm looking for a minute.
- 3x20 doorframe rows I'm looking for a minute.
- -card 48

-WORKOUT 48

MONDAY'

Backbone and Chest:

- Dip parallel in three supersets of ten repetitions, each with wide grip pull-ups. I'm looking for a minute.
- Push-ups in three supersets of ten reps with a bodyweight horizontal pull up. I'm looking for a minute.

- I am clapping push-ups in three supersets of ten reps, followed by tight grip pull-ups. I'm looking for a minute.
- Push up wide for three supersets of ten repetitions with an incline push up. I'm looking for a minute.
- abs:
- 3 x 50-second planks
- 3x15 heel touches 50 seconds of rest.

WEDNESDAY'

legs:

- Chair Leg Extension 3x15 Leg Extension 3x15 Leg Extension 3x15 Leg Extension 3x15 50 seconds of rest.
- 3 sets of 10 lunges I'm looking for a minute.
- 3x10 sumo squats I'm looking for a minute.

Shoulders:

- 3x10 pick and push up. I'm looking for a minute.
- 3 sets of 10 Hindu push-ups I'm looking for a minute.
- 3x8 burpees I'm looking for a minute.

FRIDAY'

Triceps and biceps:

- Bodyweight horizontal pull-ups in three supersets of ten repetitions with an incline push up. I'm looking for a minute.
- Pseudo plank for 50 seconds in three supersets of 10 diamond push-ups. I'm looking for a minute.
- Chin-ups in three supersets of ten repetitions, each with triceps between two benches. I'm looking for a minute.

abs:

- 3x40 seconds of side plank. 40 seconds of rest.
- 3x15 crunch 40 seconds of rest.
- -Card 49

-WORKOUT 49

- MONDAY'

Back and Chest:

- Push-ups with handles 3 supersets of 8 reps with Horizontal bodyweight pull-ups I'm looking for a minute.

- Push up on your legs in three supersets of eight repetitions of wide-grip pull-ups.
- I'm looking for a minute.
- Dip parallel three times in three supersets of the maximum amount of repetitions with tight grip pull-ups. I'm getting a minute and a half.
- Diamonds push up 3 supersets of 8 repetitions with a 40-second star plank. I'm looking for a minute.
- Push up a massive 2x15. I'm looking for a minute.

abs:

- 3x10 crunch 40 seconds of rest.

WEDNESDAY'

legs:

- 2x15 Leg Extension Chair 50 seconds of rest.
- On the step, make 3x8 lunges. I'm looking for a minute.
- Sumo squat 3x8-6-4. I'm looking for a minute.

Shoulders:

- Pick up and push up 3x8. I'm looking for a minute.
- 3x8 burpees I'm looking for a minute.
- 3x8 Hindu push-ups I'm looking for a minute.

FRIDAY'

Triceps and biceps:

- Chin up in three supersets of ten repetitions, each with dip parallel. I'm looking for a minute.
- Bodyweight horizontal chin-ups in three supersets with an incline push up. Take a minute to relax.
- Pseudo plank in three supersets of 40 seconds with diamonds push-ups for eight repetitions, followed by a minute of rest.

Abs:

- 3x30 heel taps. Take a minute to relax.
- 3x30 crunch Take a minute to relax.
- card 50

-WORKOUT 50

- MONDAY'

legs:

- 5x5 print. I'm taking two and a half minutes to recover.
- 3x8 Leg Extension I'm getting a minute and a half.
- 3x8 lunges I'm getting a minute and a half.
- 3x8 calf lift I'm getting a minute and a half.

WEDNESDAY'

Chest:

- 5x5 bench press with a barbell I'm taking two and a half minutes to recover.
- Dumbbell presses 3x8 on an incline bench set at 30 degrees. I'm getting a minute and a half.

Triceps:

- Triceps parallel with weighted 4x5 repetitions I'm taking two and a half minutes to recover.
- 3x8 cable is pushed down. I'm getting a minute and a half.

FRIDAY'

legs:

- 5x5 print. I'm taking two and a half minutes to recover.

Shoulders:

- 3x8 shoulder press I'm getting a minute and a half.

backbone:

- 4x6 lat machine I'm getting a minute and a half.

biceps:

- Curl the three-by-eight cable. I'm taking two and a half minutes to recover.
- -Card 51

TUESDAY'

Chest:

- With a 4x6 barbell, do a bench press. 2 minutes of rest.

Shoulders:

- 3x6 dumbbells for military press. I'm taking a two-minute break.

backbone:

- 3x6 rower barbell 2 minutes of rest.
- 3x6 pulley rod I'm taking a two-minute break.

Triceps:

- 3x8 French press I'm getting a minute and a half.

biceps:

- 3x8 barbell curls I'm getting a minute and a half.

THURSDAY'

legs:

- Back squats 4x6. I'm taking a two-minute break.
- 2x6 front squats I'm taking a two-minute break.
- Earth 4x6 Deadlift I'm taking a two-minute break.
- 3x8 calf sitting, I'm getting a minute and a half.
- -card 52

-WORKOUT 52

- MONDAY'

abs:

- 4 x 25 crunch 50 seconds of rest.

Chest:

- With a 4x6 barbell, do a bench press. I'm getting a minute and a half.
- Bench presses on an incline at 45' 4x6. I'm getting a minute and a half.
- The wires are crossed by 4x6. I'm looking for a minute.

backbone:

- 4x6 lat machine I'm getting a minute and a half.
- 4x6 pulley I'm getting a minute and a half.

- 4x6 rower barbell I'm getting a minute and a half.

WEDNESDAY'

legs:

- 4x6 deadlifts I'm getting a minute and a half.
- 4x6 print. I'm getting a minute and a half.
- 3x6 Leg Extension I'm getting a minute and a half.
- 3x6 Leg Curl I'm getting a minute and a half.

abs:

- 4x25 crunch 50 seconds of rest.

FRIDAY'

Shoulders:

- With a 4x6 military press. I'm getting a minute and a half.
- Risers on both sides of the 3x6 cable. I'm getting a minute and a half.

biceps:

- Recupero a minute and a half on the bench in Scott 4 x 6.
- Curl with 3x6 dumbbells. I'm getting a minute and a half.

Triceps:

- Push all the way down to the 3x6 cable. I'm getting a minute and a half.

abs:

- 4x25 crunch 50 seconds of rest.
- -Card 53

-WORKOUT 53

MONDAY'

legs:

- 5x5 print. I'm taking two and a half minutes to recover.
- Make a 3x6 cut. I'm getting a minute and a half.
- 3x6 lunges I'm getting a minute and a half.
- 4x6 calf sitting, I'm getting a minute and a half.

WEDNESDAY'

- Chest:
- 5x5 bench press with a barbell I'm taking two and a half minutes to recover.
- 4x6 dumbbell presses on an incline bench set at 30 degrees. I'm getting a minute and a half.

Triceps:

- Parallel to the triceps, 4x6. I'm getting a minute and a half.
- 4x6 cable is pushed down. I'm getting a minute and a half.

FRIDAY'

Shoulders:

- 5x5 dumbbells for the military press I'm taking two and a half minutes to recover.
- 3x8 face pulls I'm getting a minute and a half.

backbone:

- 4x6 wide grip pull-ups I'm getting a minute and a half.
- 4x6 bent over row barbell I'm getting a minute and a half.

biceps:

- 4x6 barbell curls a minute and a half of rest
- -Card 54

-WORKOUT 54

MONDAY'

Chest:

- Presses 4x8 on a flat bench. I'm getting a minute and a half.
- Dumbbell presses to 45'3x8 on an incline bench. It took me a minute and a half to recover.

Shoulders:

- 5x8 military press with dumbbells I'm getting a minute and a half.

backbone:

- Forward lat machine 3x8. I'm getting a minute and a half.

trapeze:

- 3x8 dumbbells were used to unglue. I'm getting a minute and a half.

abs:

- 3x10 overload crunch. I'm looking for a minute.

WEDNESDAY'

legs:

- 3x8 squat, I'm getting a minute and a half.
- Press size 3x8. I'm getting a minute and a half.
- 3x8 land deadlifts I'm getting a minute and a half.
- 3x8 calf sitting, I'm getting a minute and a half.

Triceps:

- 3x8 cable is pushed down. I'm getting a minute and a half.

biceps:

- 3x8 barbell curls I'm getting a minute and a half.

FRIDAY'

- Chest:
- 3x6 bench presses on a flat bench, I'm getting a minute and a half.
- 45'3x6 incline bench presses I'm getting a minute and a half.

Shoulders:

- 3x6 military press with dumbbells I'm getting a minute and a half.

- 3x6 side risers with dumbbells I'm getting a minute and a half.

backbone:

- 3x6 rower barbell I'm getting a minute and a half.

trapezius:

- 3x6 dumbbells were used to make the shake. I'm getting a minute and a half.
- Crunches with a 3x10 overload. I'm looking for a minute.
- Card No. 55

-WORKOUT 55

TUESDAY'

- Abdomen:
- 3x10 crunch I'm looking for a minute.

Chest:

- Bench press 3x8-6-4 repetitions using a barbell technical pyramid. I'm getting a minute and a half.

biceps:

- 3x8-6-4 repetitions of standing pyramidal barbell curls. I'm getting a minute and a half.

Triceps:

- 3x8-6-4 repetitions of the French Press pyramid. I'm getting a minute and a half.

Hamstrings (legs):

- 3x8-6-4 repetitions of the pyramidal leg curl. I'm getting a minute and a half.

THURSDAY'

Shoulders:

- Military press with 3x8-6-4 repetitions of a technical pyramid. I'm getting a minute and a half.

backbone:

- 3x8-6-4 pyramidal pulley repeats I'm getting a minute and a half.

legs:

- 3x8-6-4 repetitions of pyramidal horizontal press I'm getting a minute and a half.

Abdomen:

- He refused to go to the bench with a 3x10 overload. I'm looking for a minute.

- -card 56

-WORKOUT 56

- 'THURSDAY AND TUESDAY'

Chest:

- 30 'pyramidal' incline bench presses 7x12-10-8-6-10-12. I'm taking a two-minute break.

backbone:

- High pyramidal pulley 7x12-10-8-6-10-12. I'm taking a two-minute break.

legs:

- 7x12-10-8-6-10-12 pyramidal press I'm taking a two-minute break.
- In this kind of pyramidal method, the weight is gradually increased from 75% to 85/90%. (the series of 6 repetitions). Then, to finish the exercise, the weight must be reduced from 10 series of 12 repetitions.
  - card 57

-WORKOUT 57

MONDAY'

Chest:

- The 3x10 cable is crossed. I'm looking for a minute.
- Pyramidal flat push 5x8-6-4-6-8 (The load goes climbing up to the series of 4 repetitions before returning to fall in the last two sets). I'm getting a minute and a half.

backbone:

- Below a 3x10 sprocket, a sprocket one minute of rest
- 5x8-6-4-6-8 rower barbell pyramidal I'm getting a minute and a half.

WEDNESDAY'

biceps:

- 3x10 Scott bench I'm looking for a minute.
- 5x8-6-4-6-8 barbell curls with pyramidal I'm getting a minute and a half.

Triceps:

- 3x10 cables should be pushed down. I'm looking for a minute.
- Bench press with a tight grip and a pyramid method 5x8-6-4-6-8. I'm getting a minute and a half.

FRIDAY'

Shoulders:

- 3 × 10 side risers to the wires I'm looking for a minute.
- 8-6-4-6-8 military press with pyramidal 5x 8-6-4-6-8 I'm getting a minute and a half.

legs:

- 3x10 Leg Extension I'm looking for a minute.
- 5x 8-6-4-6-8 squat pyramidal s I'm getting a minute and a half.
- -Card No. 58

-WORKOUT 58

MONDAY'

legs:

- Full deadlift 6x3. 3 minutes of rest.

backbone:

- 5x5 rower barbell I'm taking two and a half minutes to recover.
- 4x6 should be pulled aside. I am taking a minute and a half Or two minutes to retrieve.

WEDNESDAY'

Chest:

- Bench press barbell with 6x3 repetitions 3 minutes of rest.
- 5x5 incline bench presses with dumbbells I'm taking two and a half minutes to recover.
- Crosses performed with 4x6 dumbbells. I'm getting a minute and a half.

FRIDAY'

- legs:
- 6x3 barbell squats 3 minutes of rest.
- 5x5 Lunges I'm taking two and a half minutes to recover.
- 4x6 Leg Curls I'm getting a minute and a half.
- -Card No. 59

-WORKOUT 59

- MONDAY'

legs:

- 5x5 squats 2 minutes recovery / 2 minutes and 30 seconds

Chest:

- Presses 5x5 on a flat bench. 2 minutes recovery / 2 minutes and 30 seconds

backbone:

- 5x5 pulley rod 2 minutes recovery / 2 minutes and 30 seconds

WEDNESDAY'

Chest:

- 4x6 parallel to the incline 1 minute and 30 seconds of rest.

backbone:

- 5x5 rower barbell 2 minutes recovery / 2 minutes and 30 seconds

Abdomen:

- Abdominals with a 4x8 overload. It's taking approximately a minute to recover.
- For one minute, do isometry from the prone position. I'm looking for a minute. Rep 4 times more.

FRIDAY'

legs:

- 5x5 deadlift land 2 minutes recovery / 2 minutes and 30 seconds

Shoulders:

- With a 5x5 military press. 2 minutes recovery / 2 minutes and 30 seconds

backbone:

- 5x5 pulley rod 2 minutes recovery / 2 minutes and 30 seconds
- -card 60

-WORKOUT 60

MONDAY'

- 6x3 bench press with a barbell (85 percent of the ceiling): two minutes and thirty seconds of rest.
- 5x5 squat (75 percent of the ceiling). I'm taking a two-minute break.
- 4x8 cut (70 percent of the ceiling). A minute and thirty seconds have been retrieved.

WEDNESDAY'

- 6x3 cut (85 percent of the ceiling). Two minutes and thirty seconds of rest.
- 5x5 barbell bench press (75 percent of the ceiling). I'm taking a two-minute break.
- 4x8 squat (70 percent of the ceiling). A minute and thirty seconds have been retrieved.

FRIDAY'

- 6x3 squat (85 percent of the ceiling). Two minutes and thirty seconds of rest.
- 5x5 cut (75 percent of the ceiling). I'm taking a two-minute break.
- 4x8 barbell bench press (70 percent of the ceiling). A minute and thirty seconds have been retrieved.
- -Card No. 61

-WORKOUT 61

TUESDAY'

Chest:

- Using a 6x5 bench press barbell, do a bench press. 2 minutes of rest.

Shoulders:

- With 6x5 dumbbells, do a military press. I'm taking a two-minute break.

backbone:

- 6x5 rower barbell 2 minutes of rest.
- 5x5 pulley rod Two minutes of rest

Triceps:

- 5x5 French Press I'm taking a two-minute break.

biceps:

- 5x5 barbell curls I'm taking a two-minute break.

THURSDAY'

legs:

- Back squats 4x5. I'm taking a two-minute break.
- 3x5 front squats I'm taking a two-minute break.
- Earth 5x5 Deadlift I'm taking a two-minute break.
- 3x8 calf sitting, I'm getting a minute and a half.
- -Card No. 62

-WORKOUT 62

MONDAY'

Chest:

- 5X4 bench press with a barbell Two and a half minutes of rest.
- Bench presses at a 45-degree angle with 5X4. Two and a half minutes of rest.

biceps:

- Chin up for a supine 5x4 grip. Two and a half minutes of rest.
- 5X4 barbell curls Two and a half minutes of rest.

Triceps:

- Recupero two and a half minutes by dipping parallel to the firm grasp 5X4.

abs:

- Crunch with an overflow of 4x8. I'm looking for a minute.

WEDNESDAY'

legs:

- 5X4 back squats Two and a half minutes of rest.
- 5X4 land deadlifts Two and a half minutes of rest.
- 3x20 calf standing, I'm looking for a minute.

FRIDAY'

- backbone:
- 5X4 pull-ups Two and a half minutes of rest.
- Dumbbells 5x4 rower Two and a half minutes of rest.

Shoulders:

* 5X4 military press Two and a half minutes of rest.
* 5X4 face pulls Two and a half minutes of rest.

abs:

* Crunch with an overflow of 4x8. I'm looking for a minute.
* -Card No. 63

MONDAY'

legs:

* 5x5 squats I'm taking two and a half minutes to recover.
* 3x8 front squats I'm getting a minute and a half.
* 3x8 lunges I'm getting a minute and a half.
* 3x8 calf lift I'm getting a minute and a half.

WEDNESDAY'

Chest:

* 5x5 barbell bench press I'm taking two and a half minutes to recover.
* Dumbbell presses 3x8 on an incline bench set at 30 degrees. I'm getting a minute and a half.

Triceps:

- 4x5 bench press with a tight grip. I'm taking two and a half minutes to recover.
- Push down on the cable 3x8. I'm getting a minute and a half.

FRIDAY'

legs:

- 5x5 deadlift land I'm taking two and a half minutes to recover.

Shoulders:

- 3x8 upright row I'm getting a minute and a half.
- backbone:
- 4x6 wide grip pull-ups I'm getting a minute and a half.

biceps:

- 3x8 barbell curls I'm taking two and a half minutes to recover.
- Card No. 64

-WORKOUT 64

MONDAY'

- legs:
- 5x5 back squats I'm taking a two-minute break.

Chest:

- 5x5 bench press with a barbell. I'm taking a two-minute break.

Triceps:

- French press with a 3x6 plate. I'm taking a two-minute break.

Abdomen:

- 5x15 crunch crunchcrunchcrunchcrunchcrunchcrunchcrunchcrun ch I'm looking for a minute.

WEDNESDAY'

legs:

- 5x5 front squats I'm taking a two-minute break.
- 5x5 deadlift land I'm taking a two-minute break.

backbone:

- 5x5 pulley rod I'm taking a two-minute break.

Abdomen:

- 5x15 crunch I'm looking for a minute.

FRIDAY'

legs:

- 5x5 print. I'm taking a two-minute break.

Shoulders:

- With a 5x5 military press. I'm taking a two-minute break.

biceps:

- 3x6 barbell curls I'm getting a minute and a half.

Triceps:

- 3x6 parallel to the incline, I'm getting a minute and a half.

Abdomen:

- 5x15 crunch crunchcrunchcrunchcrunch I'm looking for a minute.

- Card No. 65

MONDAY'

legs:

- Squat full squat 6 times. 3 minutes of rest.

back:

- Bodyweight 5x5 horizontal pull-ups I'm taking two and a half minutes to recover.
- Pull up bar 4x6. I am taking a minute and a half Or two minutes to retrieve.

WEDNESDAY'

Chest:

- 6x3 clapping push-ups 3 minutes of rest.
- 5x5 push-ups I'm taking two and a half minutes to recover.
- 4x6 parallel to the incline, I'm getting a minute and a half.
- Rotation of 4x6 planks I'm getting a minute and a half.

FRIDAY'

legs:

- 5x5 Lunges I'm taking two and a half minutes to recover.
- 4x6 side jackknives I'm getting a minute and a half.
- 4x6 slow full squats I'm getting a minute and a half.

Abdomen:

- Star Plank three times in a minute. 40 seconds of rest.
- 3x50-second side planks 40 seconds of rest.
- -card 66

-WORKOUT 66

MONDAY'

Chest:

- I am stripping 4 series on the flat bench with weight decreasing 5-5-5-20 reps. I'm getting a minute and a half.
- 3 sets of 5-5-5-20 reps of 30-degree incline bench press with stripping dumbbells. I'm getting a minute and a half.
- 2 x10 + 10 + 10 in fatigue on the incline bench to 45 degrees.
- I'm getting a minute and a half.

Shoulders:

- 4 sets of 5-5-5-20 reps of the military press with stripping dumbbells. I'm getting a minute and a half.
- In fatigue, side risers sit stripping 3 series 2 x10 + 10 + 10.

Triceps:

- I'm getting a minute and a half in French press bench press stripping 4 series with weight decreasing 5-5-5-20 reps.
- Pushdown pulldowns 2x10 + 10 + 10 till exhausted. I'm getting a minute and a half.

WEDNESDAY'

legs:

- 3 sets of 15 leg extensions. Obtain a minute.
- Squat stripping 4 series with weight going down stripping 5-5-5-20 reps I'm getting a minute and a half.
- Deadlifts 4 series, weight goes down to 5-5-5-20 reps. I'm getting a minute and a half.
- Stripping lunges 3 series with weight going down stripping 5-5-5-20 repetitions; I'm getting a minute and a half.
- 3x12 calf calfcalfcalfcalfcalf I'm looking for a minute.

FRIDAY'

backbone:

- Lat Machine or pull-free stripping 4 series with weight decreasing 5-5-5-20 repetitions I'm getting a minute and a half.
- Rower Barbell 3 sets of stripping with weight decreasing 5-5-5-20 repetitions. I'm getting a minute and a half.
- Lat Machine Tight Grip 2x6 + 6 + 6 based on availability

biceps:

- 5-5-5-20 repetitions of the barbell Curl 4 series with weight going down. I'm getting a minute and a half.
- curlscott 2x6 + 6 + 6 depending on availability
- CARD 67

-WORKOUT 67

MONDAY'

abs:

- 4x30 crunch 45 seconds of rest
- 3x10 parallel legs extended 45 seconds of rest

Chest:

- 5x6 incline bench presses I'm looking for a minute.
- The 5x6 flat bench is crossed. I'm looking for a minute.
- 3x8 + 8 + 8 stripping sequence on the flat bench I'm getting a minute and a half.

Shoulders:

- 5x6 military press with a barbell I'm looking for a minute.
- 3x10 + 10 + 10 stripping Arnold press I'm getting a minute and a half.
- Side risers superset to front raisers 3superset 10 reps for workout A minute and a half rest period between supersets.

WEDNESDAY'

- 5x6 barbell squats I'm getting a minute and a half.
- At 45 degrees, do a 5x6 press. I'm getting a minute and a half.
- 5x5 Lunges I'm getting a minute and a half.
- 3x8 + 8 + 8 leg extension stripping I'm getting a minute and a half.
- 1 x 100 repetitions of calf standing

FRIDAY'

abs:

- 4x30 crunch 45 seconds of rest
- 3x10 parallel legs extended 45 seconds of rest

backbone:

- 5x6 rower barbell I'm looking for a minute.
- 5x6 pulley I'm looking for a minute.
- Lat machine in front of 3x8 + 8 + 8 stripping. I'm getting a minute and a half.

biceps:

- 5x6 standing barbell curls I'm looking for a minute.
- Dumbbells, Curl Grip, 5x6 hammer. I'm looking for a minute.
- 3x8 + 8 + 8 curl scott stripping
- CARD NO. 68

-WORKOUT 68

MONDAY'

Chest:

- Warm up the chest press to 2x15 with a low weight. 40 seconds of rest

- Dumbbells on a 5x5 flat bench. 2 minutes of rest.
- Bench press inclination to 45'3x6. I'm getting a minute and a half.
- Crosses performed on a 3x6 incline bench. I'm getting a minute and a half.

biceps

- 4x6 barbell curls I'm getting a minute and a half.
- 3x6 curl scott, I'm getting a minute and a half.

WEDNESDAY'

legs:

- Squat four times in a row with leg extensions (4 sets of squats and leg extensions 4). In practice, you perform a set of squats for 6 reps and then transition to leg extensions for 6 reps, with a two-minute rest period in between. After resting, proceed to the next three rounds of squats and leg extensions.
- 4 supersets of deadlifts with leg curls (4 sets of deadlifts with 4 leg curl).
- The number of repetitions is 6 + 6. Two minutes are allotted for recovery.
- 3 sets of 8 calves sit. I'm regaining a minute.

FRIDAY

Shoulders:

- 2x15 heating to the shoulder press 45 seconds of rest
- 5x5 military press with barbell 2 minutes of rest.
- 3x6 face pulls I'm getting a minute and a half.
- 3x10 + 10 + 10 stripping tired Arnold press

backbone:

- Lat Machine / 4x6 broad grip pull-ups I'm getting a minute and a half.
- 4x6 rower barbell I'm getting a minute and a half.

Triceps:

- Parallel to the triceps, 5x5. 2 minutes of rest.
- Stripping depleted by 3x6 + 6 + 6 French Press.
- CARD NO. 69

-WORKOUT 69

MONDAY'

Chest:

- 4x12 repetitions of flat bench presses using barbell contrast technique. The repetitions are done with weights close to the ceiling (85 percent of maximum force), and when you are no longer able to finish the final repetition, the weight is reduced to 40% of maximum force.

- Maximum power and brings the series to a close. For example, I may perform four reps at 80 percent and then drop to 40 percent to finish the repetitions. It is critical to stimulate the muscle and potentially raise the weight or increase the number of repetitions. I am recovering for two minutes / one and a half minutes.
- Crosses performed on a 3x8 incline bench. one minute of rest
- 4x12 Incline bench lifts @ 30' with dumbbells comparison technique (4x 85 percent -45 percent). I'm taking a two-minute break.

biceps:

- 4x12 Curl Standing Contrast Method (4x80 percent - 40 percent). Recovering for two minutes / one and a half minutes.
- 3x8 curl scott curl scott curl scott curl scott curl scott I'm looking for a minute.

TUESDAY'

legs:

- 4x12 squat contrast technique (4x85 percent -45 percent). Recovering for two minutes / one and a half minutes.
- 3x8 Leg Extension I'm looking for a minute.
- 3x12 press contrast technique (4x80 percent -40 percent). I am recovering for two minutes / one and a half minutes.
- 4x15 calf sitting I'm looking for a minute.

THURSDAY'

Shoulders:

- 4x12 military press barbell comparison technique (4x85 percent -45 percent). I am recovering for two minutes / one and a half minutes.
- 3x8 side risers I'm looking for a minute.
- 3x8 face pulls. I'm looking for a minute.
- Shrugs using 3x10 dumbbells. I'm looking for a minute.

Triceps:

- The parallel bars contrast technique 4x12 (for those who perform it with a high overload) (4x80 percent -

50 percent). I am recovering for two minutes / one and a half minutes.

- 4x8 French Press I'm looking for a minute.

SATURDAY SATURDAY

backbone:

- 4x12 Chin Up Contrast Method (4x80 percent -40 percent). Recovering for two minutes / one and a half minutes.
- 3x8 rower barbell I'm looking for a minute.
- 3x12 Pulley Machine Large Contrast Method (4x80 percent -40 percent). I am recovering for two minutes / one and a half minutes.

Hamstrings (legs):

- 3x8 stiff-legged deadlifts I'm looking for a minute.
- 4x12 Leg Curl Contrast Method (4x80 percent -40 per cent). Two minutes of rest / a
- one and a half minutes
- CARD NO. 70

-WORKOUT 70

MONDAY'

Chest:

- The pectoral machine is done in three supersets, with a bench press barbell utilizing the so-called pre-fatigue approach (doing an isolated exercise immediately followed by a basic activity.) Rest two minutes.
- 3x8 parallel to the incline, I'm looking for a minute.
- Crosses on an incline bench in three supersets of ten with incline bench presses with dumbbells (the pre-fatigue technique). Rest for two minutes.

biceps:

- Curl with toe dumbbells Hammer done in three supersets of ten with sitting dumbbell curl (pre-fatigue technique). Rest two minutes.
- 3x10 curl scott, I'm looking for a minute.

TUESDAY'

legs:

- Leg extensions are performed in four supersets of ten squats with a barbell (the pre-fatigue technique). Rest for two minutes.
- Press size 3x8. I'm looking for a minute.

- 3x12 calf sitting I'm looking for a minute.

THURSDAY'

backbone:

- 5x8 pulley rod I'm looking for a minute.
- Pulley in three supersets, often with a rowing barbell (pre-fatigue technique). Rest two minutes.

Hamstrings (legs):

- Leg curls in three supersets of ten with strained leg deadlifts (the pre-fatigue technique). Rest for two minutes.

SATURDAY SATURDAY

Shoulders:

- Side risers were done in three supersets of ten military presses with dumbbells (the pre-fatigue technique). Recupero time was two minutes.
- Raise the front 3x8 inches. I'm looking for a minute.

Triceps:

- Parallel to the triceps, 3x8. I'm looking for a minute.

- French press runs in four supersets, followed by eight shoves and a bench press (opening small arms). I'm taking a two-minute break.

-card 71

MONDAY'

Chest:

- 4 × 12 barbell bench press using the rest-pause technique (The rest-pause technique is to use a weight that enables you to do 6 reps, then rest 10 seconds before starting again with the same weight and performing all the repetitions you can, then rest 10 seconds again and continue until you reach 12 repetitions.) Allow yourself two minutes of rest.
- Dumbbell crosses on an incline bench 3x8. I'm looking for a minute.
- 3x12 barbell incline presses with a rest-pause technique. I'm taking a two-minute break.

biceps:

- 3x12 rest-pause technique for barbell curls I'm taking a two-minute break.
- 3x8 curl scott curl scott curl scott curl scott curl scott I'm looking for a minute.

TUESDAY'

legs:

- 4x10 squats I'm looking for a minute.
- 3x12 Leg Extensions with Rest-Pause Method I'm taking a two-minute break.
- 3x12 print. I'm looking for a minute.
- 3x12 calf sitting I'm looking for a minute.

THURSDAY'

- 4x12 military press with rest-pause technique. I'm taking a two-minute break.
- 3x12 side raises with dumbbells sat. I'm looking for a minute.
- Raise the front 3 times using dumbbells. I'm looking for a minute.
- 4x15 dumbbells were used to create this shake. I'm looking for a minute.

Triceps:

- Parallel 4x12 using the rest-pause technique. I'm taking a two-minute break.
- 3x8 French press I'm looking for a minute.

SATURDAY SATURDAY

backbone:

- 4x12 pulley rod I'm looking for a minute.
- 3x10 rower barbell with a rest-pause technique I'm taking a two-minute break.
- 3x8 broad grip pulley machine I'm looking for a minute.

Hamstrings (legs):

- 4x8 stiff-legged deadlifts I'm looking for a minute.
- 3x10 leg curls using a rest-pause technique. I'm looking for a minute.
- -card 72

-WORKOUT 72

MONDAY'

Chest:

- Bench press for four supersets of eight reps on an incline bench set at 45 degrees. A minute and thirty seconds have been retrieved.
- Bench presses at 45' with dumbbells, 3x reps until fatigue. I'm looking for a minute.

Shoulders:

- To train with front raises, do a military press with dumbbells in four supersets of eight reps. A minute and thirty seconds have been retrieved.
- Raise one side by sitting three times through until fatigue. I'm looking for a minute.

Triceps:

- To workout with push-down, do three supersets of eight repetitions of the French Press. A minute and thirty seconds have been retrieved.
- Push-down reverse grip x 3 repetitions till tired. I'm looking for a minute.

WEDNESDAY'

legs:

- To workout with leg extensions, do four supersets of eight repetitions of barbell squats. A minute and thirty seconds have been retrieved.
- Lunges with a dumbbell or a barbell, 2x reps until exhaustion. I'm looking for a minute.
- To workout with leg curls, do four supersets of eight repetitions of deadlifts. A minute and thirty seconds have been retrieved.

- Leg curls, 2x reps until fatigue. I'm looking for a minute.
- 3x12 calf sitting I'm looking for a minute.
- 1x100 calf standing

FRIDAY'

backbone:

- Rowing with a barbell in four supersets of eight reps to work the lats.
- A minute and thirty seconds have been retrieved.
- Pulldown 3 x reps till you're exhausted. I'm looking for a minute.

biceps:

- 3x10 Traction grip strong grip supine I'm looking for a minute. (Excellent workout for both backbones and biceps.)
- 4 sets of 8 repetitions of barbell curls with curl Scott. A minute and thirty seconds have been retrieved.
    - card 73

-WORKOUT 73

MONDAY'

Back and Chest:

- 4 pyramidal series of 12-9-6-3 reps on the bench press using a barbell. I'm getting a minute and a half.
- 12-9-6-3 reps on the rower barbell in a pyramidal sequence. I'm getting a minute and a half.
- 4 supersets of 10 repetitions for each exercise:
- -Increase the slope of the bench to 30 degrees using dumbbells.
- -move the lat machine ahead
- -croci on an incline bench with dumbbells
- -handlebar pullover
- Recovery lasts 2/3 of a minute and happens after the whole superset.

WEDNESDAY'

legs:

- complete deadlift 4 pyramidal series repetitions 12-9-6-3. I'm getting a minute and a half.
- Press 4 sets of 16-13-10-7 repetitions at 45 degrees in a pyramidal sequence. I'm looking for a minute.
- 4 supersets of 10 repetitions for each exercise:
- -Lunges with dumbbells
- -extension of the legs

- -leg curling
- -A calf sits
- Recovery lasts 2/3 of a minute and happens after the whole superset.

FRIDAY'

Shoulder blades:

- 4 pyramidal series of 12-9-6-3 reps of the military press with dumbbells I'm getting a minute and a half.
- Face pulls 4 pyramidal series with repetitions of 16-13-10-7. I'm looking for a minute.

Biceps and triceps:

- 4 supersets of 10 repetitions for each exercise:
- -Standing Barbell Curl
- -triceps panca flat close grip
- -An alternating dumbbell and a curl-handle hammer
- -apply pressure on the cables
- Recovery lasts 2/3 of a minute and happens after the whole superset.
- CARD NO. 74

-WORKOUT 74

MONDAY'

Chest:

- Barbell bench press 4 sets of 5-5-5-20 reps. Rest a minute and a half.
- Incline bench presses with a 30' dumbbell, 3 sets of 5/5/20 reps. I'm getting a minute and a half.
- Crosses to the wires, 2 x reps till fatigue. I'm looking for a minute.

Shoulders:

- 4 sets of 5-5-5-20 reps of the military press with stripping dumbbells. I'm getting a minute and a half.
- 3x repeats of side risers until fatigue. I'm looking for a minute.

Triceps:

- I am stripping the French Press 4 sets of 5-5-5-20 repetitions. I'm getting a minute and a half.
- Push down to the wires twice as many times as you can till you're exhausted. I'm looking for a minute.

WEDNESDAY'

legs:

- Squat 4 sets of 5-5-5-20 repetitions. I'm getting a minute and a half.
- Dumbbell lunges, 3 sets of 3 repetitions, 05/05/20. I'm getting a minute and a half.
- Leg extension 2x reps till fatigue. I'm looking for a minute.
- 4 sets of 5-5-5-20 reps of deadlifts I'm getting a minute and a half.
- Leg curls, 2x reps until fatigue. I'm looking for a minute.
- 1x100 calf standing

FRIDAY'

dorsal:

- Lat Machine 4 sets of 5-5-5-20 repetitions. I'm getting a minute and a half.
- Pulley down with a firm grip 3 sets of repetitions 05/05/20. I'm getting a minute and a half.
- 2x reps on the rower barbell till fatigue. I'm looking for a minute.

biceps:

- Curl dumbbells for 4 sets of 5-5-5-20 repetitions. I'm getting a minute and a half.
- Curl scott 2x reps till fatigue. I'm looking for a minute.
- CARD NO. 75

-WORKOUT 75

MONDAY'

Chest:

- Three supersets:
- -6-8-10 reps of dumbbell flat press
- -Repetitions of cross-cables incline bench press 15/12/10
- I'm getting a minute and a half.
- Three supersets:
- 6-8-10 reps of incline bench press
- -Repetitions of Crosses Cables 10/12/15
- I'm getting a minute and a half.
- Triceps:

Three superseries:

- Dip the parallel with clinched elbows 6-8-10 times.
- Repetitions of the French press 10/12/15

- I'm getting a minute and a half.
- 3x12 reverse grip wires should be pushed down. I'm looking for a minute.

WEDNESDAY'

legs:

Three supersets:

- -6-8-10 reps of squat
- 12.10.15 Extension-leg reps
- I'm getting a minute and a half.
- Three supersets:
- -Stiff-legged deadlift 12 reps
- ripetiziomiripetiziomiripetiziomiripetizi
- I'm getting a minute and a half.
- 2x100 calf standing, I'm looking for a minute.
- FRIDAY'

backbone:

Three supersets:

- -Bent over rowing barbell 6-8-10 reps
- -forward 12/10/15 repetitions on the lat machine
- I'm getting a minute and a half.
- Three superseries:

* -lat Machine reversal 6-8-10 reps
* -10/12/15 repetitions with a firm hold on the pulley.
* I'm getting a minute and a half.

biceps:

Three superseries:

* -6-8-10 reps of curling the standing barbell
* 15/12/10 reps on the hammer curl
* I'm getting a minute and a half.
* I concentrated on seated curls 2x12. I'm looking for a minute.
* -Card No. 76

-WORKOUT 76

MONDAY'

Backbone and Chest:

* 4 pyramidal series 4-6-8-14 repetitions on a flat bench with a barbell. I'm getting a minute and a half.
* 4 pyramidal series of 4-6-8-14 reps on the rower barbell. I'm getting a minute and a half.
* 4 supersets of 8 repetitions on each exercise:
* -Incline bench with dumbbells to 30.'
* -move the lat machine ahead

- -crosses on an incline bench with dumbbells
- -handlebar pullover
- Recovery lasts 2/3 of a minute and happens after the whole superset.

WEDNESDAY'

- legs:
- 4 pyramidal series 4-6-8-14 reps full deadlift I'm getting a minute and a half.
- Press 4 to 45 degrees in a pyramidal sequence of 4-6-8-14 reps. I'm looking for a minute.
- 4 supersets of 8 repetitions on each exercise:
- -lunges using dumbbells
- -extension of the legs
- -leg curling
- -A calf sits
- Recovery lasts 2/3 of a minute and happens after the whole superset.

FRIDAY'

Shoulder blades:

- 4 pyramidal sequence 4-6-8-14 repetitions military press with dumbbells I'm getting a minute and a half.
- 4 pyramidal series 4-6-8-14 repetitions on the face pull I'm looking for a minute.

Biceps and triceps:

- 4 supersets of 8 repetitions on each exercise:
- -Standing Barbell Curl
- -triceps flat push tight grip
- -An alternating dumbbell and a curl-handle hammer
- -apply pressure on the cables
- Recovery lasts 2/3 of a minute and happens after the whole superset.
- -Card No. 77

-WORKOUT 77

MONDAY'

Chest:

- Bench press dumbbells in four supersets of eight repetitions to workout with crosses on an incline bench to 30'. A minute and thirty seconds have been retrieved.
- Incline bench presses @ 45' 3x6 more repetitions with the same weight until exhaustion using the rest-pause technique (10 seconds). I'm taking a two-minute break.

Shoulders:

- To train with front raises, do a military press with dumbbells in four supersets of eight reps. A minute and thirty seconds have been retrieved.

- 3x6 more reps with the same load to exhaustion with rest-pause method on the raised side by sitting 3x6 more reps with the same load to exhaustion with rest-pause method on the raised side by sitting 3x6 more reps with (10 seconds). I'm taking a two-minute break.

Triceps:

- To workout with push-down, do three supersets of eight repetitions of the French Press. A minute and thirty seconds have been retrieved.

- Push-down reverse grip 3x6 with the same weight until fatigue rest-pause technique (10 seconds). I'm taking a two-minute break.

WEDNESDAY'

legs:

- To workout with leg extensions, do four supersets of eight repetitions of barbell squats. A minute and thirty seconds have been retrieved.

- Lunges with a dumbbell or a barbell, 2x reps until exhaustion. I'm looking for a minute.
- To workout with leg curls, do four supersets of eight repetitions of deadlifts. Obtaining a
- one minute and thirty seconds
- Leg curls, 2x reps until fatigue. I'm looking for a minute.
- 3x8 calf sitting I'm looking for a minute.

FRIDAY'

backbone:

- To workout with a pull-free body, row with a barbell in four supersets of eight repetitions. A minute and thirty seconds have been retrieved.
- Pulley top 6 3x other additional repetitions with the same load to exhaustion technique with rest breaks (15.10 seconds). I'm taking a two-minute break.

biceps:

- 3x10 Traction grip strong grip supine I'm looking for a minute. (Excellent workout for both backbones and biceps.)
- 4 sets of 8 repetitions of barbell curl with curl Scott. A minute and thirty seconds have been retrieved.
- -Card No. 78

-WORKOUT 78

MONDAY'

Shoulders:

- Military press with technical pyramid repetitions of 12-8-10-6. I'm taking a two-minute break.
- 3x8 side risers plus 20 repetitions of discharge without rest, I'm getting a minute and a half.
- Raise the front three times. one minute of rest
- 3x15 side risers with a laying dumbbell I'm looking for a minute.

Triceps:

- 4x6 French Press I'm getting a minute and a half.
- 3x10 cables should be pushed down. I'm looking for a minute.

TUESDAY'

legs:

- 6x3 land deadlifts Two and a half minutes of rest.

backbone:

- 5x4 pulley rod Two and a half minutes of rest.

- Rower with 12-8-10-6 repetitions of a technical pyramid. I'm taking a two-minute break.
- Below a 3x10 sprocket, a sprocket I'm looking for a minute.

biceps:

- 3x12 curl scott, I'm looking for a minute.
- 3x8 barbell curls, followed by additional repetitions with the same weight until exhaustion using the rest-pause technique (10 seconds). I'm taking a two-minute break.

THURSDAY'

Chest:

- Bench press 12-8-10-6 reps using a barbell technical pyramid. I'm taking a two-minute break.
- 30'4x8 incline bench presses I'm getting a minute and a half.
- 3x6 parallel to the incline, I'm getting a minute and a half.
- The 3x12 cable is crossed. I'm looking for a minute.

Abdomen:

- Crunch with an overflow of 3x8. I'm looking for a minute.

- 3x60-second planks

FRIDAY'

legs:

- 12-8-10-6 repetitions of the squat pyramid method I'm taking a two-minute break.
- 3 sets of 12 lunges I'm looking for a minute.
- 3 sets of 12 leg curls I'm looking for a minute.
- 3x12 Leg Extension I'm looking for a minute.
- 3x15 calf sitting I'm looking for a minute.
- 3x30 seconds of calf standing followed by a one-minute rest.
- -Card No. 79

-WORKOUT 79

MONDAY'

Chest:

- 4 × 15 incline bench presses with dumbbells using the rest-pause technique. Recovering
- just two minutes
- 3x6 parallel to the incline, I'm taking a two-minute break.
- 3x8 dumbbell crosses on a flat bench. I'm looking for a minute.

biceps:

- 3x12 curl Scott with a rest-pause technique. I'm taking a two-minute break.
- Curl 3x8 with dumbbells while seated. I'm looking for a minute.

TUESDAY'

legs:

- 3x12 squats using a rest-pause technique, I'm taking a two-minute break.
- 3x12 Leg Extension I'm looking for a minute.
- 3x12 print. I'm looking for a minute.
- 3x25 calf sitting I'm looking for a minute.

THURSDAY'

- 4x12 military press with dumbbells using the rest-pause technique. I'm taking a two-minute break.
- With 3x12 dumbbells, lift one side at a time. I'm looking for a minute.
- 3x12 front raises retrieving a minute
- 3x15 face pulls. I'm looking for a minute.

Triceps:

- 4x6 parallel, I'm taking a two-minute break.

- 4x12 French press with rest-pause technique. I'm taking a two-minute break.

SATURDAY SATURDAY

backbone:

- 4x6 pulley rod I'm taking a two-minute break.
- 3x12 on the rower with dumbbells using the rest-pause technique. I'm taking a two-minute break.
- 3x8 broad grip pulley machine I'm looking for a minute.

Hamstrings (legs):

- 4x10 stiff-legged deadlifts I'm looking for a minute.
- 3x10 leg curls using a rest-pause technique. I'm looking for a minute.
- Card No. 80

-WORKOUT 80

MONDAY'

Chest:

- 4x12 Incline bench presses with dumbbells comparison method (4x 85 percent -45 percent). I am recovering for two minutes / one and a half minutes.

- 4x8 parallel to the incline, I'm getting a minute and a half.
- The 3x15 cable is crossed. one minute of rest

biceps:

- 4x12 curl Scott contrast technique (4x80 percent -40 percent). Recovering for two minutes / one and a half minutes.
- 3x8 barbell curl I'm looking for a minute.

TUESDAY'

legs:

- 4x12 squat contrast technique (4x85 percent -45 percent). Recovering for two minutes / one and a half minutes.
- Press size 3x8. I'm looking for a minute.
- 3x12 Leg Extension Contrast Method (4x80 percent - 40 percent). I am recovering for two minutes / one and a half minutes.
- 4x25 calf sitting I'm looking for a minute.

THURSDAY'

Shoulders:

- Military press with dumbbells vs 4x12 technique (4x85 percent -45 per cent). I am recovering for two minutes / one and a half minutes.
- 3x15, raise the front. I'm looking for a minute.
- 3x8 face pulls. I'm looking for a minute.
- Shrugs using 3x10 dumbbells. I'm looking for a minute.

Triceps:

- 4x12 French Press Contrasting Method (4x80 percent -50 percent). I am recovering for two minutes / one and a half minutes.
- Down to the 4x8 cable. I'm looking for a minute.

SATURDAY SATURDAY

- backbone:
- 4x12 rower barbell contrast technique (4x80 percent - 40 percent). Recovering for two minutes / one and a half minutes.
- 3x8 pulley rod I'm looking for a minute.
- 3x8 broad grip pulley machine I'm looking for a minute.

Hamstrings (legs):

- 3x8 stiff-legged deadlifts I'm looking for a minute.
- 4x10 Leg Curl Contrast Method (4x80 percent -40 percent). I am recovering for two minutes / one and a half minutes.

-Card No. 81

-WORKOUT 81

MONDAY'

legs:

- Make a 4x3 cut. I'm taking a two-minute break.
- backbone:
- 4 sets of 4-6-8-10 on the lat machine socket narrow pyramidal. I'm getting a minute and a half.
- 4 sets of 4-6-8-10 on the lat machine behind the pyramids. I'm getting a minute and a half.
- 3x15 latpulldowns I'm looking for a minute.

biceps:

- Curl 4 sets of 4-6-8-10 with a technical pyramid. I'm getting a minute and a half.
- Scott does a pyramidal bench press with four sets of 4-6-8-10 reps. I'm getting a minute and a half.

WEDNESDAY'

legs:

- 4 sets of 4-6-8-10 squat pyramidal s I'm taking a two-minute break.
- 3x8 lunges + 8 reps in stripping recuperation time of one and a half minutes
- 4 sets of 4-6-8-10 pyramidal press I'm getting a minute and a half.
- Leg EXTENSIONS in three super series of 12 repetitions each, followed by a two-minute rest.
- 4x15 calf sitting regaining a minute:

Abdomen:

- 3x60-second planks
- 3x15 parallel crunch. I'm looking for a minute.
- 3x30 crunch I'm looking for a minute.

FRIDAY'

Chest:

- 4 sets of 4-6-8-10 pyramidal bench press tension. I'm getting a minute and a half.
- The 3x12 cable is crossed. I'm looking for a minute.
- 4 sets of 4-6-8-10 on the pyramidal incline bench. I'm getting a minute and a half.

Shoulders:

- 3x10 Arnold press + 10 reps are stripping. I'm getting a minute and a half.
- 3x6 is sitting side risers + 6 stripping repetitions. I'm getting a minute and a half.

Triceps:

- 4x10 French Press I'm looking for a minute.
- Push all the way down to 3x6 cable + 6 + 6 stripping. I'm taking a two-minute break.
- -Card No. 82

-WORKOUT 82

MONDAY'

Chest:

- 6x8 push-ups 40 seconds of rest.
- 5x5 clapping push-ups I'm looking for a minute.
- Push up a fairly big 3x15 plot of ground. 40 seconds of rest.
- 3x20 plank rotation I'm looking for a minute.

Triceps:

- 6x8 incline pushes up 40 seconds of rest.
- 6x8 diamonds are pushed up—40 seconds of rest.

legs:

- 3 x 15 Leg Extension Chair I'm looking for a minute.
- 6x8 squat 40 seconds of rest.
- 6x8 donkey kicks 40 seconds of rest.
- On the step, make 5x5 lunges. I'm getting a minute and a half.

abs:

- 3x20 crunch I'm looking for a minute.
- 3 sets of 3 side planks. I'm looking for a minute.

FRIDAY'

back:

- Pull-up 5x5. I'm taking a two-minute break.
- 6x8 horizontal pull up bodyweight 40 seconds of rest.

Shoulders:

- 3x8 Hindu push-ups I'm looking for a minute.
- Pick up and push up 3x8. I'm looking for a minute.
- 4x8 burpees 50 seconds of rest.

biceps:

- Pseudo plank 3x maximum. I'm looking for a minute.

- -Card No. 83

-WORKOUT 83

- 'MONDAY, WEDNESDAY, AND FRIDAY'
- 1x15 is pushed up.
- Diamonds push up 1x8.
- 1x10 bodyweight horizontal pull-ups
- 1x10 pick-up and push-up
- 1 × 10 chin up
- 1x5 should be pulled up.
- 1x10 Lunges
- 1x10 squats
- 1x45 seconds of abdominal plank.
- 1x30 Cross Crunch
- 1x30 heel contact
- The circuit is completed four times. After a circuit, the recovery time is 3 minutes.
- -Card No. 84

-WORKOUT 84

- 'MONDAY, WEDNESDAY, AND FRIDAY'
- 5 minutes of aerobic exercise
- 1x10 sumo squats
- 1x10 Lunges
- 1x10 push-ups
- 1x10 pick-up and push-up

- 1x5 wide-grip pull-ups

- 1x5 jump squats

- 1x5 clapping push-ups

- 1x45 seconds of abdominal plank.

- Rep the exercises four times. After a series, the recuperation time is 3 minutes.

- Card No. 85

-WORKOUT 85

- 'MONDAY, WEDNESDAY, AND FRIDAY'

- 5 minutes of aerobic exercise

- 1x10 squats

- 1 set of 10 lunges on the step.

- 1x10 push up

- 1x10 pick-up and push-up

- 1x10 diamonds are pushed up.

- 1x10 bodyweight horizontal pull-ups

- 1x45 seconds of abdominal plank.

- Rep the exercises four times. After a series, the recuperation time is 3 minutes.

- -Card No. 86

-WORKOUT 86

- 'MONDAY, WEDNESDAY, AND FRIDAY'

- 3x15 squats I'm looking for a minute.

- 3x10 push-ups I'm looking for a minute.

- 3x15 pick-up/push-up I'm looking for a minute.

- Bodyweight 3x10 horizontal pull-ups I'm looking for a minute.
- 3x10 incline push-ups I'm looking for a minute.
- 3x30 crunch I'm looking for a minute.
- -Card No. 87

-WORKOUT 87

'MONDAY, WEDNESDAY, AND FRIDAY'

- 3 sets of 10 Lunges alternated. I'm looking for a minute.
- 3x10 push-ups I'm looking for a minute.
- 3x8 Hindu push-ups I'm looking for a minute.
- Pull-up 3x6. I'm looking for a minute.
- 3x8 diamonds are pushed up. I'm looking for a minute.
- 3x15 crunch I'm looking for a minute.
- 3x20 heel contact I'm looking for a minute.
- -Card No. 88

-WORKOUT 88

MONDAY'

Chest:

- 3 sets of 3 clapping push-ups. I'm looking for a minute.
- 3x maximum push-ups on grips with rising legs. I'm looking for a minute.

- Push uphold 3 times maximum. I'm looking for a minute.
- Maximum parallelization is 3x. I'm looking for a minute.
- 3x30 plank rotation I'm looking for a minute.

TUESDAY'

legs:

- Chair Leg Extension 1x25 Leg Extension 1x25 Leg Extension 1x25 Leg Extension 1x25
- 3x10 split squats I'm looking for a minute.
- Sumo squat 2x15 reps. I'm looking for a minute.
- Lunges on steps 5 and 5. I'm taking a two-minute break.
- 3x15 side leg lifts I'm looking for a minute.

Abdomen:

- 3x20 sitting twist I'm looking for a minute.
- 3x20 crunch I'm looking for a minute.

WEDNESDAY'

- Shoulders and back:
- Pick up and push up 3 times maximum. I'm looking for a minute.

- 3 sets of 3 Hindu push-ups with one-minute rest.
- 5x5 wide pull-up. I'm taking a two-minute break.
- 3x maximum bodyweight for horizontal pull-ups. I'm looking for a minute.
- 5x top star plank. I'm looking for a minute.

FRIDAY'

Arms:

- 4x8 chin-up bar supine I'm looking for a minute.
- Pseudo plank 4x maximum. I'm looking for a minute.
- 3x15 dips on benches (or chairs). I'm looking for a minute.
- 3x10 incline push-ups I'm looking for a minute.
- Diamonds increase the maximum by 2x. I'm looking for a minute.
- -Card No. 89

-WORKOUT 89

'MONDAY, WEDNESDAY, AND FRIDAY'

- 1x10 push-ups
- 1x30 calf standing
- Pick up and push up 1x8.
- 1x8 Hindu push-ups
- 1x10 squats

- Diamonds push up 1x8.

- 1x20 lunges

- 1x10 bodyweight horizontal pull-ups

- 1x20 bridges

- 1x1 clapping push-ups

- 1x10 incline push-ups

- 1x40 sec. Pseudo plank

- 1x30 mountain climber

- Squats on a 1x6 wall.

- 1x15 crunch

- 1x50 seconds plank

- 1x8 burpees

- 1x30 seconds of side plank.

- 1x30 bicycle crunch

- The recuperation time between circuits is one minute.

- -card 90

-WORKOUT 90

- 'MONDAY, WEDNESDAY, AND FRIDAY'

- 3x15 squats I'm looking for a minute.

- 2x15 sumo squats I'm looking for a minute.

- I am walking lunges 4x12. I'm looking for a minute.

- 2x10 wide grip pull-ups. Rest a minute.

- Pull up with a firm grip 2x10. Rest a minute.

- 3x10 push up push, so I'm looking for a minute.

- Push-ups with 4x10 diamonds I'm looking for a minute.
- 3 sets of 10 Hindu push-ups I'm looking for a minute.
- 3x10 Leg Raise I'm looking for a minute.
- 3x10 crunch I'm looking for a minute.
- 3x50-second planks I'm looking for a minute.
- -Card No. 91

-WORKOUT 91

MONDAY'

legs:

- 4x6 squat 2 minutes of rest.
- 3 sets of 8 lateral lunges. I'm getting a minute and a half.
- Front lunges 3x8. I'm getting a minute and a half.
- Donkey scores a 3x8. I'm getting a minute and a half.

Abdomen:

- 3x50-second planks I'm looking for a minute.

WEDNESDAY'

Chest:

- 5x5 clapping push-ups I'm taking two and a half minutes to recover.

- 3x8 push-ups on the legs. I'm getting a minute and a half.
- 3x15 broad push up I'm looking for a minute.

Triceps:

- 4x6 parallel to the incline 2 minutes of rest.
- 3x8 diamond push-ups I'm getting a minute and a half.

FRIDAY'

Shoulders:

- 3x8 Hindu push-ups I'm getting a minute and a half.

backbone:

- 4x6 wide grip pull-ups I'm getting a minute and a half.
- 3x8 bodyweight horizontal pull-ups I'm looking for a minute.
- biceps:
- 3x8 chin up biceps 2 minutes of rest.

Abdomen:

- 3x15 crunch I'm looking for a minute.
- -Card No. 92

-WORKOUT 92

TUESDAY'

Abdomen:

- 3x10 Russian twist I'm looking for a minute.
- 3x50-second planks I'm looking for a minute.
- 3x40 second broadside plank I'm looking for a minute.

Chest:

- 3x8-10-12 repetitions of push-ups I'm getting a minute and a half.

biceps:

- 3x8-10-12 repetitions of chin-ups I'm getting a minute and a half.

Triceps:

- Push up 3x8-10-12 repetitions with diamonds. I'm getting a minute and a half.

legs:

- Lunges on step 3 for 8-10-12 reps. I'm getting a minute and a half.

THURSDAY'

Shoulders:

- 3x8-10-12 repetitions of Hindu push-ups I'm getting a minute and a half.

backbone:

- Pull-ups with a wide grip 3x8-10-12 reps. I'm getting a minute and a half.
- legs:
- Squat 3x8-10-12. I'm getting a minute and a half.

Abdomen:

- 3x10 crunch I'm looking for a minute.
- 3x10 Leg Raise I'm looking for a minute.
- -Card No. 93

-WORKOUT 93

MONDAY'

- 3x10 split squats I'm looking for a minute.
- Chair with 3x10 leg extension. I'm looking for a minute.
- 3x10 leg side lunges I'm looking for a minute.
- 3x8 front lunges + 4 repetitions after 10 seconds rest, I'm getting a minute and a half.

- 3x15 crunch I'm looking for a minute.
- 3x10 push-ups I'm looking for a minute.
- 3 sets of 10 Hindu push-ups I'm looking for a minute.
- 3x10 bodyweight horizontal pull-ups Retrieving a minute.

THURSDAY'

- 3x10 sumo squats I'm looking for a minute.
- 3x10 bridges I'm looking for a minute.
- 3x10 Donkey kicks I'm looking for a minute.
- 3x15 reverse crunch I'm looking for a minute.
- 3x30 heel taps I'm getting a minute and a half.
- Pull-ups 3x10 I'm looking for a minute.
- 3x10 incline push-ups I'm looking for a minute.
- -Card No. 94

-WORKOUT 94

MONDAY'

- 4x15 squats I'm looking for a minute.
- 3 sets of 12 lunges on the step. I'm looking for a minute.
- 3 sets of 12 lateral lunges. I'm looking for a minute.
- 3x12 donkey kicks I'm looking for a minute.
- 3x25 crunch 30 seconds of rest.
- 3 sets of 20 bicycle crunch 30 seconds of rest.

WEDNESDAY'

- 4x12 / 10 / 8/8 push-ups I'm looking for a minute.
- Diamonds push up three times:
- 12/10/8/12/10/8/12/10/8/12/10/8/12/10/8/12/10/ 8/12/10. I'm looking for a minute.
- 3x12 pick and push up. I'm looking for a minute.
- 4 × 12/10/8/8 chin-ups I'm looking for a minute.
- 3x12 bodyweight horizontal pull-ups I'm looking for a minute.
- 3x30 heel taps 40 seconds of rest.

FRIDAY'

- 4x15 sumo squats I'm looking for a minute.
- 3 sets of 10 leg extensions I'm looking for a minute.
- 4x12 Donkey kicks I'm looking for a minute.
- 3x15 bridges I'm looking for a minute.
- 3x30 seconds of side plank. 30 seconds of rest.
- 3x40-second planks 30 seconds of rest.
- -card 95

-WORKOUT 95

'MONDAY, WEDNESDAY, AND FRIDAY'

- Running time: three minutes
- 3x20 leg extensions chair I'm looking for a minute.

- Push up between two 1x10 steps.

- 1x30 calf standing

- 1x10 pick-up and push-up

- 1x10 Hindu push-ups

- 1x10 sumo squats

- 1x8 parallel to the incline

- 1 set of 10 lunges on the step.

- 1x maximum chin up

- Donkey scores a 1x20.

- 1x1 clapping push-ups

- 1x10 dip between two benches or chairs

- 1x40 sec. star plank

- 1x15 crunch

- 1x50 seconds plank arm raise

- 1x8 burpees

- 1x30 second plank rotation

- The recuperation time between circuits is one minute.

- -Card 96

-WORKOUT 96

- MONDAY'

legs:

- 4X8-6-6-2 squat pyramidal I'm taking a two-minute break.

- Pyramidal lunges 4X8-6-6-2 I'm taking a two-minute break.

Shoulders:

- 4X8-6-6-2 Hindu push up I'm taking a two-minute break.
- Pick up the pyramidal 4X8-6-6-2 and push it. I'm taking a two-minute break.

Triceps:

- 4X8-6-6-2 pyramidal diamond push-ups I'm taking a two-minute break.

WEDNESDAY'

Chest:

- 4X8-6-6-2 push-up pyramid I'm taking a two-minute break.
- back:
- 4X8-6-6-2 pyramidal pull-up bar I'm taking a two-minute break.
- Bodyweight pyramidal horizontal pull-ups 4X8-6-6-2 I'm taking a two-minute break.

biceps:

- 4X8-6-6-2 chin-up biceps pyramid I'm taking a two-minute break.

FRIDAY'

Shoulders:

- 4X8-6-6-2 Hindu pyramidal push up I'm taking a two-minute break.

Chest:

- 4X8-6-6-2, push up 4X8-6-6-2, push up 4X8-6-6-2; I'm taking a two-minute break.

legs:

- 4X8-6-6-2 squat pyramidal I'm taking a two-minute break.

Triceps:

- The dip between two 4X8-6-6-2 chair pyramidal dips. I'm taking a two-minute break.

biceps:

- 4X8-6-6-2 biceps with elastic I'm taking a two-minute break.

- -Card 97

-WORKOUT 97

TUESDAY'

Chest:

- Push up 5 times 12-10-8-6-4. Rest a minute and a half.
- 5 X 12-10-8-6-4 push-ups with rising legs I'm getting a minute and a half.

Triceps:

- 5 X 12-10-8-6-4 dip parallel to the tight grip I'm getting a minute and a half.
- 5 X 12-10-8-6-4 push up tight opening I'm getting a minute and a half.

THURSDAY'

back:

- 5 X 12-10-8-6-4 Chins I'm getting a minute and a half.
- Bodyweight 5 X 12-10-8-6-4 horizontal pull-ups I'm getting a minute and a half.

Shoulders:

- 5 x 12-10-8-6-4 pick push-ups I'm getting a minute and a half.

quadriceps:

- 5 x 12-10-8-6-4 squats I'm getting a minute and a half.
- 5 x 12-10-8-6-4 lunges I'm getting a minute and a half.

leg:

- 3x10 sumo squats I'm looking for a minute.
- -Card 98

-WORKOUT 98

MONDAY'

Abdomen:

- 3x15 parallel crunch I'm looking for a minute.

Chest:

- 5x5 parallel dip 2 minutes of rest.
- 10x2 push-ups 3 minutes of rest.

TUESDAY'

back:

- 3x15 bodyweight horizontal pull-ups I'm looking for a minute.
- Pull up 10x2 with a broad grip. 3 minutes of rest.

WEDNESDAY'

Abdomen:

- 3x15 crunch I'm looking for a minute.

legs:

- 3x15 chair leg extension I'm looking for a minute.
- Squat 10 times on one leg. 3 minutes of rest.

THURSDAY'

Triceps:

- 4x5 diamond push-ups two minutes of recovery
- Triceps 4x5 between two chairs 3 minutes of rest.

FRIDAY'

Abdomen:

- 3x50-second planks I'm looking for a minute.

Shoulders:

- 3x5 Hindu push-ups I'm taking a two-minute break.
- Pick up and push up 10x2. 3 minutes of rest.

biceps:

- 10x2 chin up biceps 3 minutes of rest.

- -Card 99

-WORKOUT 99

MONDAY'

Chest:

- Legs 3x6 pushed up. I'm getting a minute and a half.
- 3x6 inch push-up handles I'm getting a minute and a half.
- 3x8 rotation of push-ups I'm looking for a minute.

Shoulders:

- Pick up and push up 5x6. I'm getting a minute and a half.

back:

- 3x6 chin up, I'm getting a minute and a half.
- 3x6 chins strong grip I'm getting a minute and a half.

abs:

- 3x20 plank arm raises I'm looking for a minute.

TUESDAY'

legs:

- 3x6 Split Squat I'm getting a minute and a half.

- 3x6 sumo squat I'm getting a minute and a half.
- Step 3x6 Lunges I'm getting a minute and a half.

Triceps:

- Chair with a 3x6 dip. I'm getting a minute and a half.

biceps:

- 3x6 doorframe rows I'm getting a minute and a half.

THURSDAY'

Chest:

- 3x5 push-ups of the legs. I'm taking a two-minute break.
- 3x5 push up handles I'm taking a two-minute break.
- 3x8 rotation of push-ups I'm looking for a minute.

Shoulders:

- 5x5 pick-up and push-up I'm taking a two-minute break.

back:

- 3x5 chin up broad grip I'm taking a two-minute break.
- 3x5 chin up firm grip I'm taking a two-minute break.

FRIDAY'

legs:

- 3x5 Split Squat I'm taking a two-minute break.
- 3x6 sumo squat I'm getting a minute and a half.
- Step 3x5 Lunges I'm taking a two-minute break.

Triceps:

- 3x6 dip chairs I'm getting a minute and a half.
- biceps:
- 3x6 doorframe rows I'm getting a minute and a half.

abs:

- Turkish scores 3x20. I'm looking for a minute.
- 3x20 sitting twist I'm looking for a minute.
- 3x20 plank arm raises I'm looking for a minute.
- -card 100

-WORKOUT 100

MONDAY'

Chest:

- 4 × 5 clapping push-ups Recupeo takes two minutes.
- Push your legs up and up 4 times. Recupero takes two minutes.

- Parallel dip 4x8. I'm looking for a minute.

biceps:

- 4x5 chins strong grip I'm taking a two-minute break.
- 3x50 seconds of pseudo plank. I'm looking for a minute.

abs:

- 3x12 crunch 40 seconds of rest.
- 3x12   crunch crunchcrunchcrunchcrunchcrunchcrunchcrunchcrun chcrunch 40 seconds of rest.
- Raise the legs 3x12 so that they are parallel. 40 seconds of rest.
- 3x12 heel touches 40 seconds of rest.

WEDNESDAY'

legs:

- 4x5 squats I'm taking a two-minute break.
- 4x5 lunges I'm taking a two-minute break.
- 4x8 mountain climber, I'm looking for a minute.
- 3x10 side jackknife I'm looking for a minute.

Shoulders:

- Hindu4x5 should be pushed up. I'm taking a two-minute break.
- 5x5 pick-up and push-up I'm taking a two-minute break.

FRIDAY'

back:

- Bodyweight4x5 horizontal pull-ups I'm taking a two-minute break.
- 4x5 pull-back bar I'm taking a two-minute break.
- 3x50-second star planks I'm looking for a minute.

Triceps:

- 4x5 diamond push-ups I'm taking a two-minute break.
- 3x5 Russian dip I'm taking a two-minute break.
- -card 101

-WORKOUT 101

MONDAY'

legs:

- 5x5 Jump Squat I'm taking a two-minute break.

Chest:

- Push up with 5x5 handles. I'm taking a two-minute break.

Triceps:

- 3x6 dip between two seats I'm taking a two-minute break.

Abdomen:

- 5x15 crunch I'm looking for a minute.

WEDNESDAY'

- legs:
- I am walking lunges 5x5. I'm taking a two-minute break.
- Jump 5x5 planks. I'm taking a two-minute break.

back:

- Pull-up bar 5x5. I'm taking a two-minute break.

Abdomen:

- 3 x 50-second planks 40 seconds of rest.

FRIDAY'

legs:

- 5x5 sumo squat I'm taking a two-minute break.

Shoulders:

- 5x5 pick-up and push-up I'm taking a two-minute break.

biceps:

- Pseudo plank for 3x maximum seconds. I'm looking for a minute.

Triceps:

- 3x6 parallel to the incline, I'm getting a minute and a half.

Abdomen:

- 5x15 crunch I'm looking for a minute.

Conclusion

Depending on your lifestyle, your workout plan may differ. However, to prevent injury, it is essential to practice the proper execution of the exercise.

Heating is required before each exercise. The heating time may range between 5 and 10 minutes.

Breathing should be kept under control. It inhales during the eccentric portion of the action (the descending phase) and exhales during the concentric phase (rising phase).

The cards in this list are information sheets and should not be used instead of a professional and qualified personal trainer.

The cards are a tool for expanding one's knowledge.

Fitness is more than just 30 percent exercise and 70 percent nutrition; it is also about loving your body completely.

A healthy physique will provide many advantages in your life. First, you will look more gorgeous and appealing, and you will feel more confident in yourself. Second, you'll start to grasp what it's like to battle and train hard. Finally, you will see that success comes to those that consistently train and never give up.

The key to success at the gym is to engage both your mind and your body!

Best wishes!